Healing Headaches After Brain Injury

Research-Backed Strategies for TBI, Concussion, and CTE Survivors

by

LEON EDWARD

Healing Headaches After Brain Injury

Research-Backed Strategies for TBI, Concussion, and CTE Survivors

Contents

Chapter 1:
Introduction

Understanding and managing the debilitating headaches associated with traumatic brain injuries (TBI), mild traumatic brain injuries (mTBI), concussions, and chronic traumatic encephalopathy (CTE) can feel overwhelming for survivors and their caregivers. This book is crafted to offer solace and scientifically grounded strategies to ease the path forward. By weaving through insights and practical advice on sleep, nutrition, stress, and lifestyle adaptations, the goal is to enhance the quality of life for those grappling with post-traumatic headaches.

Health professionals, too, will find this work beneficial as they seek effective management approaches for their patients. Whether you're navigating the complexities of post-injury headaches yourself or supporting someone on this journey, this book addresses the unique challenges posed by these interconnected conditions. You'll discover that the intimate ties between TBI, mTBI, concussions, and CTE, and their associated headaches, are not just statistically significant but profoundly human, underscoring the need for empathy in care.

As this journey unfolds, expect a comprehensive guide that's both enlightening and empowering, helping you understand the nuances of these conditions while providing actionable steps toward relief. Whether you are a survivor, caregiver, or healthcare provider, this resource offers tools to foster resilience and promote meaningful recovery.

Who This Book Is For

This book is designed for individuals affected by headaches following a brain injury, including traumatic brain injury (TBI), mild traumatic brain injury (mTBI), concussion, and chronic traumatic encephalopathy (CTE).

While TBI, *mTBI*, and concussion are often discussed as acute or immediate injuries caused by a single traumatic event, CTE is a neurodegenerative disease that develops over time due to repetitive brain injuries or repeated head trauma. It often affects athletes, military personnel, and others exposed to repeated head impacts. Though the symptoms of CTE, such as headaches, cognitive decline, mood disorders, and sleep disturbances, may appear years or even decades after the initial trauma, they share a strong connection with the effects of TBI, *mTBI*, and concussion.

Throughout this book, the term "brain injury survivors" will be used as an inclusive reference to encompass TBI, *mTBI*, concussion, and CTE survivors, unless a specific distinction is necessary. This approach aims to streamline terminology while ensuring clarity and inclusivity for all readers.

Headaches after brain injury present a multifaceted challenge for survivors, affecting their physical health, emotional well-being, and overall quality of life. This book is tailored to address the unique experiences and hurdles these individuals face on their journey toward recovery. Recognizing that each survivor's journey is distinct, this guide provides a nuanced understanding and practical strategies for managing headaches, a common and debilitating symptom of brain injuries.

Survivors aren't alone in their efforts to navigate life after brain injury. Family members, friends, and caregivers play an essential role in providing support and assistance. For caregivers, understanding the complexities of post-traumatic headaches can foster empathy and enable them to offer better care and support. This book serves as a resource for caregivers, equipping them with knowledge and practical tools to assist their loved ones more effectively.

Healthcare professionals, too, are part of this book's audience. Neurologists, therapists, and other specialists who treat individuals with brain injuries can find value in the comprehensive insights offered here. By delving into current research and advanced strategies for headache management, this guide provides healthcare professionals with evidence-based guidance that can enhance their practice and improve patient outcomes.

For brain injury survivors, understanding the origin and implications of their headaches can be pivotal in navigating daily life post-injury. The persistent pain or discomfort often associated with these headaches can significantly affect mood, concentration, and overall quality of life. This book's goal is to demystify the pain and provide practical steps to alleviate it. By focusing on sleep, nutrition, and stress, the guide aims to offer a holistic approach to headache management.[1]

The exploration into sleep reveals its critical role in headache management. Poor sleep can exacerbate headache symptoms, underscoring the importance of developing healthy sleep habits. This book provides survivors with tailored strategies to improve sleep quality and, consequently, manage their headaches more effectively. It discusses the importance of sleep routines that are conducive to brain health and offers tips for overcoming common sleep disturbances associated with brain injuries. Additionally, sleep disorders, such as obstructive sleep apnea and insomnia, are closely linked to headache management, and treating these sleep issues can significantly reduce headache symptoms.[2]

Nutritional considerations are another focal point in headache management. Nutrition plays a dual role: certain foods and supplements can help alleviate headaches, while others might exacerbate symptoms. This book also aims to guide readers through the intricate relationship between diet and headaches, providing actionable advice based on the latest research. Dietary changes and supplement use can offer relief for post-traumatic headaches, particularly when personalized to an individual's condition and lifestyle.[3]

Stress management, an often-underestimated factor in headache severity, is thoroughly examined in this book. Post-traumatic headaches are highly influenced by mental and emotional stress, which is why strategies such as mindfulness, meditation, and relaxation techniques are emphasized. Establishing a routine that incorporates stress-reduction strategies can break the cycle of pain and emotional tension, fostering a sense of calm and control. Biobehavioral approaches, including mindfulness-based stress reduction, cognitive behavioral therapy (CBT), and stress management techniques, have shown effectiveness in managing post-traumatic headaches by addressing both the sensory and emotional components of pain.[4]

Empowering survivors to actively participate in managing their condition is another critical focus. This empowerment is built on knowledge and self-awareness. The more informed survivors are, the better they can navigate the complexities of their symptoms and recovery process. Clear communication with healthcare professionals becomes more effective when survivors understand the dynamics of their headaches. This collaborative approach allows for the creation of personalized treatment plans tailored to their unique needs.[5]

Beyond individual strategies, community and shared experiences are powerful tools in the recovery journey. This book encourages survivors and caregivers to build a network of support—whether through local groups, online communities, or peer mentorship. Shared experiences and collective knowledge can provide emotional solace, practical advice, and a sense of belonging, which are invaluable for navigating the challenges of post-traumatic headaches.

Ultimately, this book aims to be more than just a guide—it's a companion in the recovery journey. By blending scientific research with empathetic insights, it seeks to illuminate the path forward, offering survivors, caregivers, and professionals' practical tools and emotional support to overcome the challenges of headache management after brain injury.

Note to Readers:
This book includes a mix of scientific insights, practical strategies, and personal guidance for managing headaches after brain injury. Some sections may reference medical studies, technical terms, or treatment approaches that resonate with your experiences or symptoms. If you encounter information that feels relevant to your health, we strongly encourage you to consult a qualified healthcare professional for further guidance. Personalized care based on your specific condition is essential to achieving the best outcomes.

The Impact of Headaches After Brain Injury

Headaches following a brain injury are not just simple discomfort; they can profoundly impact a person's quality of life. Whether stemming from a traumatic brain injury (TBI), mild traumatic brain injury, concussion, or chronic traumatic encephalopathy (CTE), these headaches often signify more than a mere physical ailment—they're often a daily reminder of the injury itself. This section explores how these headaches manifest and affect those who suffer, shedding light on their debilitating nature and the complex journey towards managing them effectively.

Imagine waking up in the morning and instead of feeling refreshed, your day begins with a persistent, throbbing pain. For individuals recovering from brain injuries, this scenario plays out all too frequently. The intensity and frequency of post-traumatic headaches can vary widely, affecting everything from work productivity to social interactions. What was once a simple task might become insurmountable, as the headache clouds cognitive function and drains energy reserves.

The effects extend beyond mere physical pain; emotional and psychological repercussions are deeply intertwined with chronic headaches. Anxiety and depression can compound the experience of post-traumatic headaches, creating a cycle that is difficult to break.

Those enduring these headaches often face frustration and isolation, as loved ones may struggle to comprehend their invisible battle. Many people find themselves explaining, time and again, that they are not just dealing with an ordinary headache, but a complex symptom that springs forth from the brain injury.

The prevalence of headaches after brain injury is alarmingly high. Studies indicate that up to 90% of individuals with a mild TBI report headaches within the first week post-injury, with some experiencing issues for months or even years.[6] This persistent issue highlights the critical need for effective management strategies, which this book aims to provide. Understanding prevalence helps normalize the experience and encourages sufferers to seek proper support and treatment.

It's not just the sufferers who are affected; caregivers and family members also share the burden. They often walk a fine line, wanting to offer assistance without overstepping, all while managing their own feelings of helplessness. The relentless nature of post-traumatic headaches can make social situations—and even simple family dinners—feel daunting, as the concern about triggering an attack lurks in the background. Research indicates that caregivers of TBI patients experience significant distress related to the cognitive, emotional, and behavioral changes in the injured individuals, which affects the caregivers' health and personal time. The presence of behavioral problems in TBI patients notably impacts the psychosocial functioning of caregivers, increasing their burden.[7]

Work-life balance can become precarious for those dealing with headaches post-brain injury. Concentration becomes challenging, and productivity suffers. This can lead to financial and professional instability, adding another layer of stress. For many, working remotely or changing roles may be necessary adjustments, but these shifts aren't always feasible, adding to the frustration and urgency of finding effective management strategies. Studies show that long-term recovery after TBI leads to reduced independence in areas such as employment, with many survivors requiring caregiver assistance. The cognitive, physical, emotional, and behavioral impairments post-TBI significantly impact community participation and employment, with many individuals struggling to maintain work due to ongoing symptoms. [8]

Several factors contribute to the occurrence and severity of headaches after brain injury. Neurochemical changes within the brain play a significant role post-injury, potentially altering pain pathways or even leading to the development of new, abnormal connections. Physical changes, such as tension in neck muscles or disrupted sleep patterns, can further exacerbate headaches. Often, these factors combine in complex ways that are unique to each individual, which is why a one-size-fits-all treatment rarely works.

In acknowledging the complex interplay of factors contributing to headaches post-brain injury, we can begin to appreciate why these headaches present such a formidable challenge to treat. With the intricate web of symptoms and causes, health professionals are reminded of the importance of a personalized approach to treatment plans[9] This book will review in depth strategies that encompass not just pharmacological interventions but also lifestyle adjustments, which we'll discuss in subsequent chapters.

Moreover, it's essential to acknowledge the work that caregivers and healthcare providers undertake in this space. Their compassionate support can be vital in managing the day-to-day realities of living with post-traumatic headaches. Effective treatment plans are often collaborative efforts, requiring clear communication and understanding between patient, provider, and caregiver.[10]

Despite the challenges, there's hope. Advances in research and technology continue to enhance our understanding of headaches after brain injury. This growing body of knowledge offers promising avenues for new treatments and management strategies, leading to better outcomes for sufferers. As we continue exploring various approaches, it is vital to remain proactive and adaptable, as what's effective today may evolve with future discoveries.

Finding effective management strategies for headaches after brain injury is crucial not only for relieving physical pain but also for improving overall quality of life. By addressing the root causes and understanding the far-reaching implications, we can better equip ourselves to handle these challenges. This book aims to offer guidance and support through practical, research-backed strategies designed to empower readers on their journey to recovery and headache management.

As we move forward, we'll explore the types of headaches associated with brain injuries, the science behind their development, and the numerous ways they can be effectively managed. Armed with knowledge, survivors and their supporters can work together to optimize care strategies, mitigate symptoms, and foster environments conducive to healing and improved well-being.

Understanding the Connection Between TBI, mTBI, Concussion, CTE, and Headaches

Traumatic Brain Injuries (TBIs), mild TBIs (mTBIs), concussions, and Chronic Traumatic Encephalopathy (CTE) are terms commonly encountered in discussions surrounding sports injuries, accidents, and military service. While all involve injury to the brain, their causes, outcomes, and symptom presentations often differ. Despite these differences, headaches are a pervasive and debilitating symptom linking these conditions, significantly affecting the quality of life of those who endure them.

The relationship between TBIs, mTBIs, concussions, CTE, and headaches stems from the brain's vulnerability to trauma. A TBI refers to any disruption of brain function caused by external force, and it can range in severity from mild to severe. Mild TBIs (mTBIs), which often overlap with concussions, are characterized by brief changes in mental status or consciousness but may present with persistent symptoms, including headaches.[11]

Concussions, often considered a subset of mTBIs, result from biomechanical forces to the head or body that cause the brain to move within the skull, or from a direct blow to the head or violent shaking. While concussions typically involve transient neurological impairment, they can trigger a cascade of biochemical changes leading to persistent and debilitating headaches.[12]

In contrast, CTE is a progressive neurodegenerative disease caused by repetitive head trauma. Unlike TBI or concussion, which often result from a single traumatic event, CTE develops gradually from repeated brain injuries or repeated impacts over time. It is most commonly diagnosed posthumously in athletes, military personnel, and others exposed to chronic head trauma. CTE symptoms, including chronic headaches, often appear years or even decades after the trauma and typically progress alongside cognitive and emotional changes.[13]

The mechanisms underlying these headaches vary across conditions but often involve inflammation, disruptions in cerebral blood flow, and nociceptive pathway activation, such as trigeminal sensitization.[14] Trauma-induced imbalances in neurotransmitters like serotonin and dopamine further contribute to the persistence of headaches, particularly tension and migraine types.

In addition to physiological factors, emotional and psychological elements play a significant role. Stress, anxiety, and depression, often secondary to brain injuries, can intensify headache symptoms, creating a feedback loop that exacerbates both mental health challenges and headache frequency.[15]

Understanding the interconnectedness between physiological and psychological factors is crucial for effectively managing headaches after a brain injury. Clinical insights, combined with patient-reported outcomes, provide a comprehensive perspective, highlighting the importance of early identification of headache patterns and triggers post-injury. A multimodal approach to treatment—including medication, lifestyle adjustments, and supportive therapies—often proves most effective. Emerging research highlights the role of nociceptive pathways, particularly trigeminal sensitization (sometimes described in the literature as increased trigeminal nociceptive activity), in the acute emergence of post-traumatic headaches, shedding light on potential mechanisms that may inform targeted interventions.[16]

Early identification of headache patterns and triggers post-injury is vital for effective management. Treatment strategies should adopt a multimodal approach, combining medication, lifestyle adjustments, and supportive therapies. Emerging research on the brain's plasticity highlights its capacity for recovery, underscoring the importance of tailored interventions that address each individual's unique experience.[17]

Healthcare professionals working with individuals affected by TBIs, mTBIs, concussions, and CTE face the dual challenge of addressing both the physical and psychological components of these conditions. By integrating personalized care, they can provide meaningful relief to patients grappling with the multifaceted burden of post-traumatic headaches.

As research continues to evolve, our understanding of the pathways linking brain trauma to chronic headaches will deepen, potentially unveiling novel therapeutic approaches. For now, a holistic and compassionate approach remains the cornerstone of effective management, empowering survivors and fostering resilience in the face of adversity.

What to Expect: A Guide to This Book

Embarking on a journey towards managing headaches after brain injury, this book serves as a comprehensive guide for those affected by traumatic brain injury (TBI), mTBI, concussion, or chronic traumatic encephalopathy (CTE), as well as their caregivers and healthcare professionals. Understanding the nuances of these conditions is no small feat. "What to Expect: A Guide to This Book" provides a roadmap for readers to navigate the chapters ahead, setting the stage for a meaningful and purposeful exploration. This section aims to outline the primary components of the book, offering insights into the various strategies and knowledge that await.

Starting with Chapter 1, the "Introduction" sets the tone by elucidating the challenges faced by individuals dealing with headaches post-brain injury. It establishes who the book is meant for and discusses the profound impact these headaches have on daily life. The connection between TBIs, concussions, CTE, and headaches is explored, helping readers understand the interwoven nature of these conditions. The introduction also highlights the empathetic, research-backed approach this book embraces, focusing on tangible improvements in quality of life.

As readers progress to Chapter 2, they will delve into the intricacies of different headache types, including tension-type headaches, migraines, and post-traumatic headaches. This chapter offers insightful distinctions between the symptoms and triggers specific to TBI, concussion, and CTE survivors. Recognizing when to seek professional help is emphasized, empowering readers to make informed decisions about their health.

Chapter 3 focuses on understanding mild traumatic brain injury (mTBI) and its specific implications for headaches. Unlike other forms of brain injury, mTBI presents unique challenges, particularly regarding persistent headaches and subtle neurological changes that require tailored approaches. Readers will gain insights into headache patterns linked to mTBI, alongside strategies for identifying triggers and exploring management options. The significance of seeking professional assistance when necessary is also underscored.

Chapter 4 delves into the scientific mechanisms behind headache development after brain injuries, exploring the neurological and physiological changes that occur post-injury. Drawing from recent research, this chapter provides a foundational understanding to support effective management strategies..

To aid in self-awareness and proactive health management, Chapter 5 introduces the concept of tracking headache patterns. Readers learn about the value of maintaining a headache diary, capturing details such as frequency, intensity, and potential triggers. By identifying patterns, individuals can make more informed treatment choices. The chapter also reviews various tools and apps designed to assist in monitoring headaches.

Chapter 6 shifts focus to the "Role of Sleep in Headache Management." Recognizing how sleep impacts headache severity and frequency allows readers to develop brain-healthy sleep routines. Practical tips for overcoming sleep disturbances are shared, aligning with the book's holistic approach to headache management. Emphasis is placed on fostering restorative sleep to facilitate overall wellness.

Moving on to Chapter 7, readers gain insights into "Nutrition for Headache Relief." The book examines foods that can either exacerbate or alleviate headaches. The critical role of hydration in headache prevention is also highlighted. Leveraging research-backed nutritional strategies, including supplements that may aid in headache reduction, offers another avenue for improvement.

Chapter 8 explores stress management techniques, illustrating the impact of stress on post-traumatic headaches. Highlighting mindfulness, meditation, and relaxation techniques, the chapter guides readers towards developing effective stress-reduction routines. The goal is to equip individuals with tools that can mitigate the adverse effects of stress and foster a sense of calm and control.

The benefits of physical activity are discussed in Chapter 9. It outlines safe exercises tailored for TBI and concussion survivors, emphasizing how physical activity can reduce headache frequency. Balancing activity levels to avoid overexertion is crucial, ensuring that exercise remains a supportive rather than aggravating factor in headache management.

For those seeking deeper insight into conventional treatments, Chapter 10 examines the spectrum of medical treatments and interventions available for post-traumatic headaches. From commonly used medications to alternative therapies such as physical therapy, the chapter highlights the importance of collaborating with healthcare professionals for customized treatment solutions.

The book's practical approach continues with Chapter 11, which focuses on lifestyle adjustments for headache prevention. Readers learn how to create daily routines conducive to minimizing headache occurrences by identifying and avoiding personal triggers. Building a supportive environment for recovery is also explored, promoting a holistic lifestyle change.

Chapter 12 emphasizes the value of building a solid support system, which is crucial for lasting recovery. Readers are encouraged to seek support from family, friends, and caregivers. Effective communication of personal needs is discussed, as well as finding and joining support groups or online communities where shared experiences foster understanding and camaraderie.

Finally, Chapter 13 ties everything together by guiding readers in creating a holistic headache management plan. This chapter integrates elements such as sleep, nutrition, physical activity, and stress management, stressing the importance of customizing a plan geared towards long-term relief. Readers are encouraged to take an active role in their recovery, empowering themselves through informed decision-making and strategic planning.

The conclusion of the book reiterates key takeaways while providing encouragement for ongoing adaptation and managing headaches after brain injury. This chapter serves as a reminder of the proactive steps readers can take in their journey towards improved well-being, reinforcing the tools and strategies discussed throughout the book.

While this book is structured to be read from cover to cover, it is also designed to accommodate those seeking specific information. With a thoughtfully curated flow, navigating from one section to another is seamless for both in-depth understanding and targeted reference. Whether you're navigating the content as a survivor seeking actionable relief, a caregiver looking for insights, or a professional searching for evidence-based strategies, this book is designed to adapt to your needs

Chapter 2:
Understanding Headache Types

Navigating life after a traumatic brain injury often means dealing with a variety of headaches, including tension-type, migraines, and post-traumatic headaches. Each type presents distinct symptoms that affect individuals differently. Tension-type headaches, for example, may feel like a tight, squeezing band around the head, whereas migraines can cause intense pain accompanied by nausea and light sensitivity. Recent research highlights that headaches post-TBI are not only common but can become chronic if not managed effectively.[18] Comprehensive treatment approaches now emphasize a combination of lifestyle modifications, physical therapy, and medication, underscoring the importance of early intervention.[19] Additionally, tension-type headaches are frequently underdiagnosed and often mislabeled as migraines due to overlapping symptoms.[20]

Post-traumatic headaches, particularly after mild traumatic brain injury (mTBI), present unique challenges due to their prevalence and variability. Up to 90% of mTBI patients experience headaches, with tension-type headaches being the most common subtype. In military populations, however, migraines dominate as the primary complaint. Individuals with a premorbid history of primary headaches, particularly females, may be more susceptible to persistent post-traumatic headaches.[21] While this chapter provides an overview of these headache types and their overlapping characteristics, readers seeking an in-depth exploration of mTBI-specific headache challenges are encouraged to refer to Chapter 3: Understanding Mild Traumatic Brain Injury and Headaches for further insights.

Tension-Type Headaches, Migraines, and Post-Traumatic Headaches

Recognizing the nuances between tension-type headaches, migraines, and post-traumatic headaches is crucial for individuals living with the aftermath of a traumatic brain injury (TBI), concussion, or chronic traumatic encephalopathy (CTE). Each type presents distinct characteristics that can significantly affect one's quality of life and approach to treatment. Understanding these differences forms the foundation for effective headache management strategies tailored to those who have experienced brain injuries.

Tension-type headaches are among the most common headache forms globally. For someone who has experienced a brain injury, including mTBI, these headaches often manifest as a pressing or tightening sensation around the head. Unlike migraines, tension-type headaches do not typically involve the severe nausea or visual disturbances known as auras. Despite their ubiquity, the exact pathophysiology behind tension-type headaches remains a topic of ongoing research, with some studies suggesting links to muscular and psychological stress factors.[22]

While tension-type headaches are more about persistent dull pressure, migraines introduce a whole different level of intensity. Migraines typically feature a throbbing or pulsating pain, often on one side of the head, and can last from a few hours to several days. They frequently come with a constellation of symptoms, such as nausea, vomiting, and sensitivity to light and sound. For survivors of TBI and mTBI, migraines may be exacerbated by sensory overload or stress, which can be more challenging to manage post-injury.

Post-traumatic headaches are particularly relevant to this audience, as they are directly tied to brain injuries. Such headaches tend to mirror the characteristics of tension-type or migraine headaches but are exacerbated by the trauma itself. In individuals with mTBI, post-traumatic headaches are frequently reported as a primary symptom, often persisting for weeks or months following the injury. The mechanisms by which brain injuries give rise to these headaches are still under investigation, with current research pointing towards dysregulation in the brain's pain processing centers and inflammatory pathways.[23] Readers seeking a deeper exploration of mTBI-specific headaches will find expanded insights in Chapter 3.

For healthcare professionals assisting in the management of these headaches, distinguishing between these types is essential for choosing the most appropriate therapeutic interventions. Tension-type headaches might respond better to nonsteroidal anti-inflammatory drugs (NSAIDs), whereas migraines often require triptans or prophylactic medications like beta-blockers or antidepressants. Post-traumatic headaches, particularly after mTBI, may benefit from a combination of pharmacological and non-pharmacological approaches, emphasizing the need for personalized treatment plans.

Certain lifestyle changes can significantly ease all three headache types. Regular physical activity tailored to the individual's capacity serves as both a preventive measure and an alleviator of symptoms. In particular, gentle exercises like walking, yoga, or swimming help maintain physiological well-being without straining the brain. These activities can stimulate endorphin release and promote better sleep patterns, which are both beneficial in headache management.[24]

Nutritional adjustments also play a vital role. A balanced diet rich in anti-inflammatory foods such as omega-3 fatty acids, found in fish and nuts, can reduce headache frequency and severity. Adequate hydration is equally important; even mild dehydration can precipitate headaches, particularly in those already dealing with post-traumatic symptoms. Caffeine management is critical as well; it can offer relief in some cases but may contribute to rebound headaches if consumed excessively.

Stress management offers another layer of control over headache symptoms, especially in the context of post-traumatic headaches. Techniques such as mindfulness and meditation can provide profound benefits by reducing overall stress levels and improving mental resilience. Stress often acts as a trigger, and by learning to navigate it more effectively, individuals can significantly decrease the frequency and intensity of their headaches.

While exploring these non-pharmacological strategies, collaboration with healthcare professionals remains key. Patients should feel empowered to communicate openly about the effectiveness of treatments and any side effects they might experience. A multidisciplinary approach that includes neurologists, physiotherapists, and even psychologists or counselors could provide the comprehensive care needed for managing post-traumatic headaches effectively.

Incorporating a holistic headache management plan not only involves addressing the immediate symptoms but also enhancing the overall quality of life. Those living with the aftermath of brain injuries —including mTBI, TBI, and CTE— need to feel supported both medically and socially, as understanding the interplay between headache types and personal circumstances can lead to more empathetic and effective care.

Ultimately, the journey to managing these headaches is personal and multifaceted. By grasping the distinctions between tension-type headaches, migraines, and post-traumatic headaches, individuals and caregivers can unlock a path to tailored strategies that foster recovery and enhance well-being.

Symptoms and Triggers Specific to TBI, mTBI, Concussion, and CTE Survivors

The complex interplay between traumatic brain injuries (TBI), concussions, mild traumatic brain injuries (mTBI), and chronic traumatic encephalopathy (CTE) with headaches creates unique challenges in recovery and daily life. These conditions introduce distinct symptoms and triggers that differ from those associated with common tension-type headaches or migraines. Understanding these nuances is key to effective management and improving quality of life.

Survivors often report persistent headaches that vary widely in intensity and type, ranging from constant throbbing pain to sharp, stabbing sensations. These headaches may not emerge immediately after the injury but can develop weeks or even months later, creating ongoing frustration and uncertainty. Commonly associated symptoms, such as heightened sensitivity to light and sound, often compound the discomfort, making normal activities difficult to manage. Cognitive challenges like impaired memory or reduced concentration may further intensify the impact of headaches, presenting an additional layer of difficulty.[25]

Triggers for these headaches can be highly individualized and, at times, unpredictable. While external factors such as bright lights, loud noises, or certain smells may provoke symptoms in some, others might find emotional stress, anxiety, or depression to be significant contributors. Physical triggers like neck tension or excessive physical exertion are also common, particularly among mTBI and concussion survivors. These triggers can fluctuate over time, influenced by the unique physiology of the injury and evolving circumstances.[23]

Post-traumatic headaches are often part of a self-reinforcing cycle. Headaches may disrupt sleep, which in turn increases headache susceptibility. Sleep disturbances, a frequent issue for TBI, mTBI, and concussion survivors, exacerbate symptoms and delay recovery. Similarly, dehydration or irregular eating habits can amplify headache intensity, highlighting the importance of balanced nutrition and hydration as part of an effective management strategy.[26]

For caregivers and healthcare providers, it's essential to recognize that symptoms and triggers can vary significantly between individuals. The presence of comorbid conditions, such as post-traumatic stress disorder (PTSD), can intensify headaches, creating a need for integrated care plans that address both mental and physical health. Understanding the interconnected nature of these factors is vital for designing effective, personalized treatment strategies.

Open communication with healthcare providers is crucial in managing these symptoms and triggers. While medications such as NSAIDs, triptans, or prophylactic drugs may offer relief, non-pharmacological interventions often play an equally significant role. Cognitive-behavioral therapy, mindfulness practices, and stress management techniques have been shown to provide meaningful benefits in reducing headache frequency and intensity.[27]

Maintaining a headache diary remains a powerful tool for identifying personal patterns and triggers. By documenting the frequency, intensity, and potential contributing factors of headaches, survivors and their care teams can develop tailored strategies that address specific needs. Tracking this information over time also provides insights into the effectiveness of various treatments, fostering a more responsive and adaptable management plan.[28]

This section provides a foundation for understanding the broader context of symptoms and triggers related to TBIs, concussions, and CTE. Readers interested in exploring triggers and tailored management specific to mTBIs will find an in-depth discussion in Chapter 3. Together, these chapters offer a comprehensive framework for addressing the varied and complex challenges of post-traumatic headaches.

By combining scientific research with empathetic strategies, survivors and caregivers can navigate recovery with greater confidence. Embracing a multifaceted approach that includes medical interventions, lifestyle adjustments, and psychological support paves the way for meaningful progress and lasting relief.

When to Seek Professional Help

Headaches following traumatic brain injury (TBI), concussion, mild traumatic brain injury (mTBI), or chronic traumatic encephalopathy (CTE) can be challenging to navigate. They aren't just routine discomforts to endure; they can be debilitating and often require professional attention. While some headaches are expected post-injury, there comes a point where navigating them alone becomes ineffective or even risky. Knowing when to seek assistance from healthcare professionals is essential to ensure proper treatment and management..

The first key indicator that you should seek professional help is the frequency of headaches. If you're experiencing headaches more days than not, or if they seem to be increasing in frequency, it's time to reach out. Chronic post-traumatic headaches are a known complication of TBI and mTBI, often requiring customized treatment plans to manage effectively.[29] Healthcare professionals can assess the pattern and frequency of your headaches to guide treatment decisions and potentially prevent them from becoming a chronic condition.

Severity is another crucial element to consider. If the intensity of your headaches frequently scales toward the severe end, significantly impairing your ability to carry out daily tasks, it's essential to consult a healthcare provider. Severe headaches, particularly following an mTBI, may indicate underlying issues requiring immediate attention. Medical professionals can evaluate clinical characteristics and associated conditions to provide tailored interventions that address both the intensity of the pain and its impact on daily functioning.[30]

In addition, if your headaches are accompanied by neurological symptoms, such as visual disturbances, weakness, confusion, loss of balance, or personality changes, it's crucial to seek immediate medical evaluation. These symptoms could suggest a more severe condition requiring urgent medical intervention. Neurologists and mental health professionals specializing in post-traumatic injuries can conduct comprehensive evaluations, integrating psychological support and therapeutic strategies to manage these headaches effectively.[31]

Persistent headaches are another red flag. If headaches persist despite lifestyle adjustments, stress management, and over-the-counter medications, professional consultation is warranted. Lingering headaches can affect emotional well-being and exacerbate other post-concussive symptoms, further delaying recovery. Healthcare professionals can intervene with medication adjustments, therapy, or alternative treatments to provide relief.[32]

Sometimes, identifying headache triggers proves elusive despite thorough self-management efforts. This is especially common in mTBI cases, where headache patterns may overlap with or mimic other conditions. Healthcare providers can assess the clinical characteristics and comorbidities, using diagnostic tools to develop individualized treatment plans. This comprehensive approach is particularly beneficial for mTBI patients, who often experience complex interactions between physical and emotional symptoms influencing headache patterns.[30]

Emotional factors cannot be overlooked. If headaches contribute to emotional distress or mental health declines, it's another reason to seek medical advice. For example, individuals with mTBI may experience heightened emotional sensitivities or post-traumatic stress disorder (PTSD), which can exacerbate headaches. Integrated treatment approaches addressing both emotional and physical symptoms are essential in such cases.[32] Mental health professionals collaborating with neurologists can combine psychological support with traditional headache treatments for holistic care.[31]

Including family members and caregivers in medical consultations is another important consideration. Engaging them in understanding the complexities of mTBI and other brain injuries equips them to provide more effective support. Healthcare providers can guide caregivers in fostering environments that minimize headache triggers and support recovery. This collaborative approach not only improves headache management but also enhances emotional and physical outcomes for survivors.

Suppose you find yourself overwhelmed by the impact of headaches—whether they strain professional responsibilities, personal relationships, or overall well-being. In that case, professionals trained in managing post-traumatic conditions can offer tailored interventions to reclaim functionality and improve quality of life.

Professional help is a vital resource in addressing post-traumatic headaches. While self-management strategies are essential, recognizing when to seek intervention ensures optimal care and minimizes the risk of complications. Whether you're dealing with headaches post-TBI, concussion, mTBI, or CTE, connecting with healthcare professionals provides the expertise necessary to regain control over your recovery journey. With the assistance of neurologists, headache specialists, mental health experts, and a supportive network, effective headache management is within reach.

Chapter 3:
Understanding mTBI and Its Impact on Headaches

Mild traumatic brain injury (mTBI), often resulting from events like sports injuries or minor falls, carries profound implications for those affected, especially concerning headaches. Characterized by a temporary disruption of brain function, mTBI often leads to headaches that can be puzzling due to their variability and persistence. Common headache types associated with mTBI include tension-type headaches and migraines, each presenting unique challenges in terms of management and impact on daily life. These headaches stem from neurological changes and physiological disruptions within the brain, amplifying sensitivity to triggers like light, noise, and stress. Understanding these factors is crucial for individuals and healthcare providers as they navigate tailored management strategies, which may encompass both medical and alternative interventions. With mTBI headaches having such a substantial impact on quality of life, recognizing when to seek professional help can make all the difference in effective care. Moreover, education and support can empower survivors to advocate for themselves in the vast landscape of treatment options, creating pathways to improvement.[33],[34],[35]

Defining mTBI and Its Characteristics

Mild traumatic brain injury, frequently abbreviated as mTBI, is often referred to as a concussion in medical and public discourse. This type of injury results from a blow or jolt to the head, leading to temporary disruptions in brain function, such as changes in mental status or consciousness. While symptoms of mTBI can vary widely among individuals, they generally reflect a transient disturbance in normal brain activity. Despite being labeled "mild," the implications of mTBI should not be underestimated, as they can significantly affect daily life, particularly in the form of persistent headaches.[36] These challenges emphasize the importance of understanding the condition's complexity and addressing it with appropriate care.

When comparing mTBI with moderate or severe traumatic brain injuries (TBIs), the primary distinction lies in the extent of damage and potential for long-term impairment. Moderate to severe TBIs often result in extended periods of unconsciousness or amnesia, along with observable structural damage on imaging scans such as MRI or CT. Conversely, mTBI typically does not present with visible structural changes on standard imaging, which can lead to the misconception that it is inconsequential. However, mTBI can still result in significant functional impairments, including prolonged headaches and cognitive difficulties, which impact quality of life long after the initial injury.[37] This highlights the need for comprehensive evaluation and tailored management strategies.

It is also crucial to differentiate mTBI from concussions and chronic traumatic encephalopathy (CTE). While all concussions fall under the category of mTBIs, not all mTBIs meet the clinical criteria for a concussion. Concussions are typically characterized by acute symptoms that resolve relatively quickly with rest and proper care. In contrast, mTBIs may involve more complex and persistent symptoms that require longer recovery periods. Meanwhile, CTE represents a degenerative brain condition associated with repeated head trauma, commonly observed in athletes and military personnel. Unlike mTBI or concussion, CTE is typically diagnosed posthumously and is linked to long-term symptoms such as memory loss, behavioral changes, and progressive neurological decline. Recognizing these distinctions is key to providing accurate diagnosis and effective care.

Understanding Symptoms and Prevalence

The hallmark symptoms of mTBI often encompass a combination of physical, cognitive, and emotional challenges. Physical symptoms, such as persistent headaches, dizziness, and heightened sensitivity to light or noise, are among the most commonly reported issues. These physical symptoms often coexist with cognitive difficulties, including memory impairment, confusion, and challenges with concentration. Emotional disturbances, such as irritability, anxiety, and depression, can exacerbate the impact of physical and cognitive symptoms, creating a compounded effect on an individual's quality of life.[38]

In terms of prevalence, mTBI is one of the most frequently occurring neurological disorders, often resulting from incidents such as sports injuries, falls, motor vehicle accidents, and workplace accidents. According to studies, up to 80% of individuals with mTBI experience headaches during the initial recovery phase, making headaches one of the most persistent and debilitating consequences of the injury[39]. Furthermore, for many survivors, these headaches do not resolve in the short term and may persist for months or even years, presenting a significant barrier to full recovery and functional independence.

Understanding these prevalence trends and the pervasive nature of headaches following mTBI helps establish the importance of early intervention and targeted management strategies. Identifying patterns in symptom persistence, such as recurring headaches triggered by sensory overstimulation or emotional stress, is critical to formulating effective treatment plans. As subsequent sections will explore, tailoring these strategies to address the unique needs of each individual can lead to more meaningful and sustainable improvements in quality of life

Common Headache Types Associated with mTBI

Headaches are a frequent and often debilitating complaint following a mild traumatic brain injury (mTBI). Their varied presentation and intensity can significantly burden the recovery process. Understanding the types of headaches associated with mTBI is crucial for developing effective management strategies. The most prevalent headache types include post-traumatic headaches, tension-type headaches, and migraine-like headaches, each presenting unique characteristics and triggers.

Post-Traumatic Headaches

Post-traumatic headaches are among the most commonly observed in individuals recovering from an mTBI. These headaches are classified based on the timeline of their occurrence: acute or chronic. Acute post-traumatic headaches typically develop immediately after the injury or within the first week and resolve within three months. Chronic post-traumatic headaches persist beyond this period, often requiring more complex and long-term management strategies.[40] This transition to chronicity underscores the need for early intervention and tailored treatment plans to prevent symptoms from becoming entrenched.

Tension-Type Headaches

Tension-type headaches are another prevalent form observed in mTBI survivors. These headaches are characterized by a diffuse, pressing pain that can feel like a tight band around the head. Stress and muscle tension are primary triggers, and individuals recovering from an mTBI may be particularly susceptible due to both the physical and emotional aftereffects of their injury. The increased stress of managing the consequences of mTBI, combined with heightened sensitivity to muscular tension, often exacerbates these headaches.[41] Addressing both the physical and psychological factors contributing to tension-type headaches is critical to their management.

Migraine-Like Headaches

Migraine-like headaches are also common among mTBI survivors, often presenting as a pulsating pain accompanied by light sensitivity, nausea, and occasionally visual disturbances. These symptoms closely resemble those of classic migraines, making them particularly debilitating for individuals during recovery. Environmental factors such as bright lights or loud noises and hormonal fluctuations are common triggers that can amplify the severity of migraine-like symptoms. For mTBI survivors, managing these triggers is often essential to improving their quality of life.[42]

Psychological and Emotional Impacts
The complexity of dealing with post-mTBI headaches extends beyond their physical manifestation. The unpredictability and persistence of these headaches can lead to emotional challenges, including frustration, anxiety, and even depression. These psychological impacts, in turn, may worsen the severity or frequency of headaches, creating a vicious cycle. Identifying underlying stressors and adopting targeted interventions can help survivors break this cycle, reducing headache severity and improving overall mental health.

Tailored Management Strategies
Each headache type associated with mTBI requires a nuanced, individualized approach to management. While pharmacological treatments like NSAIDs or triptans may alleviate symptoms, addressing underlying triggers is equally critical. Lifestyle modifications, such as regular physical activity, stress management practices, and adjustments to environmental factors, play a vital role in preventing headaches and reducing their frequency. Collaboration with healthcare providers is essential to tailor a comprehensive strategy that addresses both physical and psychological aspects of headaches. With the right combination of interventions, survivors of mTBI can achieve significant relief and enhance their overall quality of life.

Neurological and Physiological Impacts of mTBI

Mild traumatic brain injuries (mTBI) can have a profound impact on the brain's physical and neurological functions, leading to significant complications such as headaches. When someone experiences an mTBI, it often results in subtle yet impactful disruptions in neural networks—these are the pathways the brain utilizes to communicate internally and process information.

Changes in these complex networks can provoke the onset of headaches by disrupting the brain's normal processing and messaging functions.[43]

In addition to neural disruptions, mTBI can alter blood flow and increase inflammation in the brain. These physiological changes contribute to headache development due to the brain becoming oxygen-starved or inflamed tissues exerting pressure on surrounding structures, leading to pain sensations.[44] The brain's unique environment in the aftermath of an mTBI can thus become a breeding ground for chronic headaches if left unaddressed.

Headaches after mTBI aren't just about physical changes within the brain; sensory sensitivities also play a crucial role. Many individuals with mTBI report heightened sensitivity to light, sound, and smell, making them more susceptible to headache triggers. This increased sensitivity results from the brain's compromised ability to filter and manage environmental stimuli after an injury.[45] For instance, ordinary stimuli such as fluorescent lighting, loud conversations, or strong odors, which would typically be unnoticeable, can become sources of discomfort and contribute to escalating headache intensity. Understanding and managing these sensory triggers is essential for developing effective headache management strategies. Tools such as tinted glasses, noise-canceling headphones, or air purifiers can help alleviate the impact of these triggers, offering survivors greater comfort and adaptability in everyday environments.

Understanding these sensory sensitivities is key to managing post-mTBI headaches. They don't merely cause headaches, but also exacerbate existing headache symptoms, making everyday environments potentially overwhelming. Strategies to mitigate these effects often involve creating low-stimulation environments or adopting tools such as tinted glasses and noise-canceling headphones to ease the burden on the brain.[43]

Research into the neurological and physiological impacts of mTBI is continuously evolving. Recent studies have explored how subtle changes in neural connectivity post-mTBI can serve as predictors for long-term headache experiences, providing insights into more personalized treatment approaches.[44] These studies hint at a future where mTBI-induced headaches might be managed more effectively, with healthcare providers tailoring interventions to the specific neurological changes present in each individual.

Moreover, emerging research focuses on the role of inflammation in post-mTBI headache persistence. By understanding the inflammatory processes that occur after a brain injury, scientists hope to develop targeted anti-inflammatory treatments that could alleviate headaches and improve recovery outcomes.[45] As this body of research grows, it promises new therapies that directly address the neurological dysfunctions specific to mTBI.

The insights garnered from these studies also emphasize the importance of early intervention in mTBI cases. Initiating treatment shortly after an injury might prevent the neurological and physiological changes that contribute to post-traumatic headaches from becoming entrenched. Such an approach could pave the way for better long-term quality of life for those affected.[43]

Ultimately, the neurological and physiological impacts of mTBI are complex, with each individual's experience being influenced by a variety of factors. Effective headache management hinges on understanding these intricacies and recognizing that mTBI not only alters brain function but also affects sensory perceptions and overall brain health. Through ongoing research and tailored management strategies, it's possible to mitigate these impacts, offering hope and practical pathways for those affected by mTBI-induced headaches [44].

This understanding positions healthcare professionals and caregivers to better support mTBI survivors, fostering environments and adopting techniques that acknowledge both the visible and hidden impacts of mTBI on headache experiences. An empathetic and scientifically informed approach can make a significant difference in the lives of those navigating the complexities of life after a brain injury.

Continued research and increased awareness about the intricate workings of mTBI will be pivotal in shaping future headache management practices. By aligning caregiving strategies with scientific advancements and patient insights, it may soon be possible to minimize headache occurrences and facilitate improved recovery journeys for mTBI survivors.[45]

Identifying Triggers and Tailored Management

Understanding what sparks headaches in individuals with mild traumatic brain injuries (mTBI) requires a keen awareness of the common triggers and an exploration of personalized management strategies. Each survivor's experience is unique, making it essential to identify specific elements that exacerbate their symptoms. By doing so, survivors and their caregivers can more effectively manage the frequency and intensity of post-injury headaches.

Many mTBI survivors notice headaches are tied to sensory overload, such as bright lights or loud noises. The brain's increased sensitivity after injury can turn routine stimuli into unbearable triggers. Survivors often avoid busy environments, such as shopping centers or concerts, to prevent headaches. Poor sleep is another culprit. When sleep patterns are disrupted, whether from difficulty falling asleep or frequent waking, headache occurrences can increase. Establishing a consistent sleep schedule can therefore play a crucial role in headache management.[46]

Stress and Headaches: Stress, too, plays a significant part in provoking post-traumatic headaches. The body's response to stress can lead to muscle tension and vascular changes that contribute to headache pain.[47] When stress levels rise, the brain's pain pathways can become hypersensitive, resulting in increased headache frequency and severity. To effectively minimize stress-triggered headaches, incorporating relaxation techniques such as deep breathing exercises, meditation, or yoga into daily routines is beneficial. This not only helps in alleviating immediate stress but also builds long-term resilience. Engaging in regular physical activities like walking or swimming can further help regulate stress hormones and improve overall mental well-being. As the American Migraine Foundation emphasizes, relaxation therapy and structured stress management techniques, such as stress inoculation training, can play a critical role in mitigating headache frequency and severity.[48]

Hydration is crucial in reducing headache frequency. Dehydration can contribute significantly to headache development, yet it's often overlooked. Ensuring adequate fluid intake throughout the day is a manageable step toward headache reduction. Some mTBI survivors might require more personalized hydration plans due to varying activity levels or other health conditions.[49]

Physical activity, when approached carefully, serves as a beneficial management strategy. While overexertion can act as a trigger, gentle exercises tailored to the individual's recovery progress can mitigate headache symptoms. Activities like walking, swimming, or light stretching promote better circulation and release endorphins, which are natural painkillers for the body. The key is to balance activity with rest, ensuring that exercise does not lead to fatigue or increased headache intensity.

Pacing Daily Activities: Pacing daily activities proves essential in avoiding symptom exacerbation. It's important for survivors to plan their day to include breaks, allowing the brain time to rest and recover.[47] Structured rest periods can prevent the accumulation of fatigue, which is a known trigger for headaches. This approach helps in managing energy levels and reduces the risk of triggering headaches from accumulated fatigue. Techniques such as time management strategies and setting realistic goals for daily tasks can support this pacing. Additionally, using tools like planners or reminder apps can help individuals stay organized and ensure they take regular breaks throughout the day. The Ontario Neurotrauma Foundation highlights the value of tracking activities to identify triggers and of implementing cognitive and physical pacing strategies as essential components of headache management.[50]

Identifying triggers and tailoring management strategies not only reduce the occurrence and severity of headaches but also enhance the survivor's quality of life. Collaborating with healthcare professionals can lead to developing a customized plan that incorporates these strategies, ensuring a comprehensive approach to management.

Although the journey to identifying triggers may require patience and perseverance, the rewards in terms of headache management and improved daily function are significant. Keeping an open line of communication with caregivers and health professionals is also crucial. Together, they can navigate the complexities of mTBI recovery, crafting a supportive environment that addresses the individual needs and concerns of the survivor.

By dedicating time to understand personal headache patterns and triggers, mTBI survivors can become more proactive in their recovery process. This proactive stance fosters empowerment and encourages a holistic approach to managing post-traumatic headaches, integrating physical, emotional, and environmental adjustments to sustain long-term improvements.

Medical and Alternative Interventions

Understanding how to manage headaches associated with mild traumatic brain injury (mTBI) requires delving into both medical and alternative interventions. These headaches are not just a nuisance; they can severely impact one's quality of life. A holistic approach that combines established medical treatments and alternative therapies offers the best hope for relief. In this section, we'll explore some of these interventions and how they can be effectively utilized.

Among medical approaches, medications are often the first line of defense against mTBI-related headaches. Neurologists and primary care providers frequently prescribe a range of medications tailored to the specific type and severity of the headache. Common classes include non-steroidal anti-inflammatory drugs (NSAIDs), triptans, and, in certain situations, anticonvulsants or antidepressants, which have proven effective in managing headaches.[51] Some individuals may find significant relief through these medications, though it's crucial for patients and caregivers to be aware of the potential side effects and the importance of medical supervision.

Cognitive-behavioral therapy (CBT) emerges as a noteworthy non-pharmacological medical intervention. CBT aids in changing negative thought patterns and behaviors that contribute to headache severity and frequency. By focusing on the psychological aspects of headache management, CBT empowers patients to develop coping strategies that reduce both anxiety and the perception of pain.[52] This method can be particularly beneficial for those whose headaches are exacerbated by stress or mood issues, making it an essential component of a comprehensive headache management plan.

In recent years, there has been a growing interest in alternative therapies for headache relief, especially among those who seek non-medication options or wish to complement their existing treatments. Acupuncture is one such therapy, rooted in traditional Chinese medicine, which involves inserting thin needles into specific body points to balance the body's energy flow. Research suggests that acupuncture can effectively reduce the frequency and intensity of headaches by promoting endorphin release and enhancing circulation, offering a safe treatment option with relatively few side effects.[53]

Biofeedback is another increasingly popular alternative intervention. This technique involves using electronic monitoring to convey information about physiological activities, such as heart rate and muscle tension. By learning to control these physiological processes through relaxation and visualization techniques, individuals can reduce headache severity over time. Biofeedback provides a tangible way to understand the connection between stress and physical symptoms, which is beneficial for managing mTBI-related headaches.[54]

Mindfulness practices, including meditation and yoga, foster a state of heightened awareness and relaxation, which can be transformative for headache sufferers. Engaging in regular mindfulness exercises helps break the cycle of pain and stress that often exacerbates headaches. By focusing on the present moment and reducing anxiety, mindfulness contributes not only to headache relief but also to overall well-being.[55] By incorporating these practices into a daily routine, individuals often find they can better manage their symptoms and improve their quality of life. These techniques, while particularly beneficial for mTBI survivors, are equally effective for those living with other forms of brain injuries, including TBI and CTE. For detailed exercises and practical applications, readers are encouraged to explore the section on mindfulness and relaxation in Chapter 8, which offers actionable strategies tailored for diverse needs.

For individuals experiencing sensory sensitivities post-mTBI, desensitization therapy could be a valuable part of treatment. These sensitivities can manifest as light, sound, or even touch-induced pain or discomfort, which often trigger or worsen headaches. Desensitization therapy involves gradually exposing individuals to these triggers in a controlled manner to reduce their sensitivity and the associated impact on headache frequency.[56] This therapy helps patients reclaim their environments and activities, further supporting their recovery journey.

Integrating these medical and alternative interventions isn't merely about finding a one-size-fits-all solution. It's about creating a personalized approach that addresses the unique needs of each individual. Collaboration between healthcare providers and patients is essential in crafting a tailored plan that considers medical history, preferences, and lifestyle. By actively participating in their healthcare journey, patients can explore what combination of therapies provides them the most relief and leads to a significant improvement in their daily lives.

Ultimately, the journey to managing mTBI-related headaches involves trial, perseverance, and often a blend of interventions. While some may find relief quickly, others may need time to discover what works for them. Nonetheless, the landscape of medical and alternative interventions offers a wealth of options to explore. Continuing research and innovation in this field suggest hope for even more effective strategies in the future.

When to Seek Professional Help

Living with the consequences of a mild traumatic brain injury (mTBI) can be daunting, particularly when it leads to persistent headaches. While self-management strategies and lifestyle modifications can help alleviate some discomfort, there are times when professional intervention is necessary. Recognizing the signs that warrant a deeper level of care is essential for ensuring a better quality of life and preventing further complications.

One of the most critical red flags indicating the need for professional assistance is worsening headaches. After an mTBI, it's normal to experience headache episodes; however, if you notice a significant increase in intensity or frequency, it might indicate an underlying issue that requires medical evaluation.[57] Additionally, accompanying symptoms such as vision changes or severe dizziness can further complicate the situation, making it even more urgent to consult a healthcare provider. These symptoms might suggest increased intracranial pressure or other complications that need timely intervention.

Emotional fluctuations are another critical aspect to monitor. Changes in mood, including irritability or anxiety, are common following an mTBI, but persistent or worsening emotional disturbances might suggest more significant concerns like depression or anxiety disorders. The psychological impact of chronic headaches and the frustration of delayed healing can significantly affect mental health.[58] If you or your loved one experiences prolonged bouts of sadness or a loss of interest in previously enjoyed activities, seeking help from a mental health professional can be a crucial step towards recovery.

Building a multidisciplinary care team can provide a comprehensive approach to managing the complex symptoms associated with mTBI. Neurologists play a pivotal role in this team, often taking the lead in diagnosing and managing post-traumatic headache disorders. They can prescribe medications and recommend interventions that align with your individual needs.[59] Physiatrists, specialists in physical medicine and rehabilitation, complement the neurologist's efforts by creating tailored rehabilitation programs designed to improve both physical and cognitive functions affected by the injury. These programs can also help address persistent headache triggers and enhance overall well-being.

To further enhance recovery, physical therapists contribute movement-based therapeutic interventions aimed at alleviating musculoskeletal issues often linked to headaches, such as neck and shoulder tension. These therapists develop safe exercise routines that enhance blood flow, promote relaxation, and reduce pain.[60] Depending on the specific circumstances, the care team might also include occupational therapists to assist with daily activities and psychologists to address the emotional impacts of mTBI.

Understanding when to seek professional help is vital for anyone navigating the challenges of mTBI-related headaches. By promptly addressing physical and emotional red flags and leveraging the expertise of a multidisciplinary team, you can take significant steps toward relief and recovery. Acknowledging the need for professional support demonstrates a proactive approach to health management, leading to more effective symptom management and an improved quality of life after a brain injury

Chapter 4:
The Science of Headaches and Brain Injury

Introduction

Understanding how brain injuries lead to the development of headaches involves exploring intricate neurological and physiological changes. When the brain experiences trauma, such as a TBI, concussion, or mTBI,, the initial impact can cause direct physical damage to brain tissues and blood vessels. This damage disrupts the normal regulation of cerebral blood flow and triggers a cascade of biophysical and biochemical responses as the brain attempts to repair itself. These responses often include inflammation, oxidative stress, changes in the brain's neurovascular functioning, and alterations in neurotransmitter levels, which can all contribute to the onset and persistence of headaches.[61],[62]

Understanding the Pain Pathways: Neurogenic Inflammation and Nociceptive Processing

Following a brain injury, the body responds in ways that can lead to chronic headaches. One critical response involves the disruption of nociceptive pathways—these are the networks responsible for detecting and processing pain signals. This disruption, known as dysfunction in nociceptive processing, alters how pain signals are transmitted and regulated within the brain.[63]

In brain injury cases, including those resulting from TBI, mTBI, concussion, or CTE, these pathways can become hypersensitive, leading the brain's natural systems for pain control to overreact to otherwise mild or normal stimuli. This hypersensitivity often involves the release of neuropeptides like calcitonin gene-related peptide (CGRP), which contributes to neurogenic inflammation. Neurogenic inflammation causes swelling and increased sensitivity to pain due to nerve inflammation, a process that can significantly exacerbate headaches.[64]

For individuals with brain injuries, including those resulting from TBI, mTBI, concussion, or CTE, understanding these disruptions in nociceptive pathways is crucial. What might begin as transient or mild pain signaling can transform into persistent and debilitating headache syndromes. This neurogenic inflammation plays a central role in prolonging headaches, making recovery and daily life more challenging. By recognizing the relationship between brain injury, disrupted nociceptive pathways, and headaches, healthcare providers and survivors can better tailor treatment strategies that address these specific pain mechanisms, leading to more targeted and effective relief.

How Brain Injuries Lead to Headache Development

Headaches following a brain injury are more than just a side effect; they are often a direct consequence of complex processes within the brain. The shock from a traumatic brain injury (TBI), concussion, or mTBI sets off a cascade of physiological and neurological changes. Let's explore the mechanisms that transform an injured brain into one prone to discomfort and pain.

The Body's Healing Response and Inflammation

After a brain injury, the body initiates biochemical and cellular processes aimed at healing. However, this response often also triggers headaches. Inflammation is one of the primary culprits. When the brain experiences trauma, it triggers an inflammatory response to repair damaged tissues. While inflammation is essential for healing, it can cause swelling and increased pressure in the head, leading to headaches.[65]

Research by Dennis et al. found that the body's natural inflammatory response after brain injury, while aimed at healing, can inadvertently increase pressure and sensitivity in the brain, setting the stage for headaches. In brain injury survivors, including those recovering from TBI, mTBI, concussion, or CTE, diffuse inflammation can sometimes persist longer than expected, exacerbating symptoms like headaches and cognitive fatigue.

The Role of Neurotransmitters in Pain Sensitivity

The nerves and blood vessels within the brain are highly sensitive to changes in pressure and inflammation. Post-injury, neurotransmitters like substance P and calcitonin gene-related peptide (CGRP) are released in greater quantities. These messengers can cause blood vessels to dilate, contributing to headache symptoms by altering pain pathways and increasing sensitivity.[66]

This dysregulation of neurotransmitters is common among brain injury survivors, including those recovering from TBI, mTBI, concussion, and CTE. Many survivors report heightened sensitivity to light, sound, and stress as key headache triggers, underscoring the role of neurotransmitter imbalances in post-injury pain sensitivity.

Disrupted Neural Functioning and Pain Perception

Brain injuries often disrupt normal neural functioning, particularly in areas like the thalamus and brainstem that regulate pain processing. These disruptions result in abnormal pain perception, leaving survivors more sensitive to headache triggers and environmental stimuli.[67] Advanced neuroimaging has shown that damage to these circuits, alongside psychological factors such as stress and anxiety, can intensify pain processing, emphasizing the need for targeted therapeutic approaches.

Advanced neuroimaging has shown that damage to these circuits, alongside psychological factors such as stress and anxiety, can intensify pain processing, emphasizing the need for targeted therapeutic approaches.

Axonal injury, a common outcome of brain injuries—including TBI, mTBI, concussion, and CTE—further exacerbates these issues by disrupting the brain's communication pathways. This damage, as

Kim et al. explain[68] , stems from complex biomechanical forces that contribute to persistent headaches and neurological deficits.

By understanding how these pathways are affected, survivors and healthcare providers can better address the root causes of headache persistence, paving the way for more effective management strategies. combining both medical and holistic approaches.

Blood Flow and Oxygenation Challenges

Brain injuries can disrupt normal blood flow and oxygenation, a critical challenge post-TBI or concussion. Following such injuries, the brain's energy demand increases sharply due to neurotransmitter release and ionic imbalances, leading to an "energy crisis" as ATP supplies become inadequate.[69] This cascade not only strains oxygen and glucose availability but also initiates an inflammatory response, increasing the brain's vulnerability to secondary injuries. As the brain adapts to this metabolic stress, such disruptions can lead to headaches and other persistent symptoms, underscoring the need for a gradual, carefully monitored recovery.

The Psychological Impact: Stress and Anxiety

Brain injuries don't only cause physiological changes; they also introduce emotional and psychological disturbances that can intensify headache experiences. Stress and anxiety are common among brain injury survivors, including those recovering from TBI, mTBI, concussion, or CTE. These psychological disturbances are closely linked with headache severity, compounding the physical burden of recovery. This underscores the need to address both physical and psychological consequences of brain injury in headache management.[70]

Unpacking the Complexity of Post-Traumatic Headaches

Considering these factors, it becomes clear why headaches are a frequent companion post-brain injury. They're the result of a combination of blood flow anomalies, chemical imbalances, and an impaired nociceptive (pain-processing) system—each compounding to create persistent pain and discomfort. For some individuals, these headaches become chronic or persistent, aligning with a condition known as Persistent Post-Traumatic Headache (PTH).[71;72]

Persistent PTH is increasingly understood as a multifactorial condition, in which neuropathic pain pathways become hypersensitive after an injury, leading to an exaggerated pain response.[72] This hypersensitivity, combined with altered brain connectivity in regions responsible for pain processing, makes persistent headaches a challenge for many brain injury survivors, including those recovering from TBI, mTBI, concussion, or CTE.

Understanding this complexity highlights the necessity for targeted treatments that address multiple factors, such as reducing inflammation, regulating neurotransmitters, and managing stress.

Hope for Future Treatments and Precision Medicine

As research progresses, new insights into the mechanisms of persistent post-traumatic headaches are emerging. Studies now suggest that **precision medicine** approaches—treatments customized to target specific biological and neurological pathways disrupted by TBI—may hold promise in offering relief for those suffering from PTH. Personalized interventions based on individual pain profiles, including techniques to manage neuropathic pain sensitivity, could represent a new frontier in headache management.[73,74]

With a multifaceted approach targeting the unique combination of disrupted pathways in each patient, precision medicine offers hope for effective, long-lasting relief. For healthcare providers and brain injury survivors alike, a focus on comprehensive, individually tailored treatments may pave the way to improved outcomes and quality of life.

Importance of Understanding Headache Origins

Understanding the origins of headaches after brain injury, is crucial for guiding effective management strategies. Persistent post-traumatic headaches (PTH) often arise from complex interactions between neurological, psychological, and physiological factors. These factors may include neurogenic inflammation, disrupted pain pathways, and emotional stressors. Treatment plans can be tailored to address specific mechanisms at play—such as reducing inflammation, regulating neurotransmitter activity, and managing stress and anxiety. This multifaceted approach is essential for addressing the unique challenges faced by survivors. The intersection of neurology, psychology, and medicine offers a powerful framework for developing comprehensive headache management strategies, ensuring that treatment is grounded in a holistic understanding of these conditions.[72,73]

Personalized Headache Management Strategies

Recognizing the unique nature of each individual's experience with headaches post-brain injury is vital for effective care. For survivors of brain injuries, regular consultations with healthcare professionals and close monitoring of headache patterns help ensure that treatment plans are tailored to their specific needs. Personalized strategies that combine medical, psychological, and lifestyle approaches—such as addressing sleep, nutrition, and stress—form the foundation of long-term headache relief. By actively collaborating with healthcare providers and leveraging tools like headache diaries, survivors can better understand their triggers and work towards sustained recovery. This individualized approach is essential for achieving meaningful improvements in both headache management and overall quality of life.

Neurological and Physiological Changes Post-Injury

When a brain injury occurs, whether classified as a traumatic brain injury (TBI), concussion, chronic traumatic encephalopathy (CTE), or mild traumatic brain injury (mTBI), it triggers a complex cascade of neurological and physiological changes. These disruptions are central to understanding the pathophysiology of headaches and offer insights into management and therapeutic strategies tailored to the type of injury.

Inflammation: A Double-Edged Sword

The brain's inflammatory response is one of its first defenses against injury. While inflammation aids in repairing damaged tissues, excessive or prolonged inflammation can increase intracranial pressure and heighten sensitivity, contributing to headache persistence.

This dual role of inflammation is particularly significant in brain injury survivors, including those recovering from TBI, mTBI, concussion, or CTE, where neuroinflammation may not always manifest visibly on imaging but can still lead to chronic symptoms like headaches.[75]

Recognizing and addressing inflammation early is crucial to mitigating long-term effects and reducing headache persistence.

Blood-Brain Barrier Disruption

Injury to the brain can compromise the blood-brain barrier (BBB), a critical structure that regulates the brain's internal environment. When the BBB's integrity is disrupted, foreign substances may infiltrate, exacerbating inflammation and affecting pain pathways. This process is associated with persistent headaches across all types of brain injuries.[76]

Axonal Injury and Signal Disruption

Diffuse axonal injury (DAI), common in TBI and occasionally present in mTBI and concussion, disrupts the brain's neural signaling pathways.[77] This damage can lead to protein accumulation, neuronal death, and persistent headaches.

For brain injury survivors, including those recovering from TBI, mTBI, and concussion, axonal injuries may not be detectable through standard imaging but can still significantly impact pain perception, cognitive function, and recovery.[78]

Neurotransmitter Shifts

Post-brain injury, neurotransmitter levels such as serotonin and dopamine often become imbalanced, impacting mood, cognition, and pain perception. These shifts are closely linked to headache development in survivors of mTBI, TBI, and concussion. Addressing these changes through pharmacological or behavioral interventions can be pivotal for recovery.[79]

Neural Reorganization and Pain Processing

The brain undergoes reorganization after an injury, particularly in the central and autonomic nervous systems. This restructuring often involves hyperactivity in pain pathways, including those associated with the trigeminal nerve, leading to increased headache frequency and intensity. This phenomenon is observed across the spectrum of brain injuries, underscoring the need for advanced diagnostic and treatment approaches.[80]

Hormonal Imbalances

Injuries affecting the hypothalamic-pituitary axis (HPA) can result in hormonal fluctuations, contributing to fatigue, mood disturbances, and headaches. This disruption is most prevalent in moderate-to-severe TBI cases, where damage to the HPA is more pronounced.

However, survivors of mTBI or concussion, particularly those with prolonged symptoms, may also experience subtle hormonal imbalances that significantly affect their quality of life. Recognizing and addressing these disruptions through hormonal therapies may play a critical role in comprehensive headache management plans.[81]

Vestibular System Disruptions

The vestibular system, responsible for balance and spatial orientation, is often affected by brain injuries of varying severities, including TBI, mTBI, and concussion. Disruptions to this system can result in symptoms such as dizziness, vertigo, nausea, and balance difficulties, which are commonly reported across all brain injury types. For some survivors, these symptoms are particularly triggered by visual motion sensitivity or environments with excessive motion, such as crowded spaces or rapidly changing visual stimuli.

Concussions and Vestibular Symptoms:

Research highlights that mild brain injuries, including concussions, frequently involve vestibular dysfunction, often due to subtle disruptions in the brainstem and inner ear pathways. Symptoms like lightheadedness, vertigo, and difficulty with coordination are prevalent in concussion survivors, particularly when visual motion sensitivity is present.[82]

Moderate-to-Severe TBI and Vestibular Symptoms:

While vestibular disruptions are common in concussions and mTBI, they can be more pronounced in moderate-to-severe TBI survivors due to the potential for structural damage to the brainstem, cerebellum, or inner ear. Survivors of more severe injuries often report persistent or debilitating symptoms, which may include chronic dizziness, profound imbalance, and visual-vestibular integration deficits.[83]

Variability of Severity Across Brain Injuries:

It's important to note that symptom severity doesn't always correlate directly with the injury's classification (e.g., mild vs. severe). For example, mTBI or concussion survivors with prolonged symptoms may experience significant vestibular dysfunction, even in the absence of structural damage detected on imaging.[84]

Conversely, survivors of severe TBI may show recovery in vestibular symptoms earlier if other rehabilitation factors are optimized.

Treatment and Recovery:

Vestibular rehabilitation therapy (VRT) has proven effective in addressing these symptoms for all brain injury survivors. Tailored exercises to improve balance, gaze stabilization, and motion tolerance can significantly enhance recovery and quality of life, particularly for those with persistent symptoms.

Oxidative Stress and Cellular Damage

Brain injuries generate oxidative stress through free radical accumulation, leading to cellular damage and inflammation. These mechanisms are common across brain injuries, including TBI, mTBI, concussion, and CTE, and contribute to persistent headache symptoms.

Antioxidants and neuroprotective agents may help mitigate these effects, offering relief from symptoms such as headaches and fatigue. This avenue may be particularly relevant for survivors with prolonged symptoms, such as those recovering from mTBI or concussion, who could benefit from tailored dietary or pharmacological interventions.[85]

Psychological Impact: Stress and Anxiety

The psychological consequences of brain injuries—such as stress, anxiety, and depression—often exacerbate headache conditions. These effects can create a feedback loop of discomfort and emotional distress, where persistent headaches contribute to worsening mood disturbances and vice versa.

For brain injury survivors, including those recovering from TBI, mTBI, concussion, or CTE, breaking this cycle is critical. Counseling and integrative therapies can help address the emotional and psychological impacts of brain injury, providing a holistic approach to symptom management.[86]

Toward a Personalized Approach in Headache Management

Each individual's response to brain injury is unique, influenced by the severity of the injury, pre-existing conditions, and personal health. Personalized headache management strategies that address these neurological and physiological changes are essential for improving outcomes. For brain injury survivors, including those recovering from TBI, mTBI, concussion, or CTE, tailoring treatment to the specific disruptions and challenges they face offers hope for long-term recovery and relief.[87]

Future Directions: Advancements in Imaging and Biomarkers

Emerging technologies, such as advanced imaging and biomarker identification, are revolutionizing the study of headaches associated with brain injuries. Functional MRI and blood-based biomarkers are uncovering the intricate relationships between injury severity and persistent symptoms, offering pathways to more precise and effective treatments.[88] Continued research into these areas holds promise for all brain injury survivors, including those with mTBI, TBI, concussion, or CTE.

Insights from Recent Research

Recent research has significantly advanced our understanding of the links between headaches and brain injuries, including traumatic brain injury (TBI), concussion, chronic traumatic encephalopathy (CTE), and mild traumatic brain injury (mTBI). Headaches are a common consequence of these injuries, and their underlying mechanisms and effective management strategies remain active areas of study. These insights are pivotal for improving the quality of life for survivors and their caregivers by paving the way for more effective treatments.

Neuroinflammation and Headaches

The Dual Role of Inflammation

Recent research has significantly advanced our understanding of the links between headaches and brain injuries, including traumatic brain injury (TBI), concussion, chronic traumatic encephalopathy (CTE), and mild traumatic brain injury (mTBI). Headaches are a common consequence of these injuries, and their underlying mechanisms and effective management strategies remain active areas of study. These insights are pivotal for improving the quality of life for survivors and their caregivers by paving the way for more effective treatments.[75]

Therapeutic Targets in Neuroinflammatory Pathways

Research supports targeting neuroinflammatory pathways as a promising therapeutic approach for PTH management. Interventions focused on modulating inflammation could mitigate chronic headaches and offer new avenues for treatment

Summary:

- Neuroinflammation is a key factor in the development of PTH.

- Targeting inflammatory pathways can mitigate chronic headaches.

- Balancing inflammation is essential for effective treatment.

Neurotransmitter Alterations

Serotonin and Dopamine Dysregulation

Alterations in neurotransmitter systems, particularly serotonin and dopamine, are linked to post-traumatic headaches (PTH). Serotonin dysregulation, a key factor in migraine pathogenesis, also underlies many post-traumatic headache mechanisms observed across brain injury survivors, including those recovering from TBI, mTBI, and concussion.

Pharmacological Interventions
Studies indicate that pharmacological modulation of these neurotransmitter systems could provide effective treatments for PTH, with potential application across TBI severity levels.[89]

Summary:
- Dysregulation of serotonin and dopamine contributes to PTH.

- Pharmacological modulation offers new treatment strategies.

Brain Connectivity and Imaging Studies

Functional MRI Findings
Advances in imaging studies, such as functional MRI (fMRI), have highlighted structural and functional brain changes following injuries. Disruptions in connectivity within brain networks, especially those involving the thalamus and cortical areas, are prevalent in persistent headache cases across brain injury survivors, including those recovering from TBI, mTBI, and concussion.[90]

Summary:
- Altered brain connectivity contributes to persistent headaches.

- fMRI studies help identify specific neural pathways involved in PTH.

Genetic Predispositions

Genetic Markers and Headache Susceptibility
Genetic predispositions play a significant role in the susceptibility and severity of post-traumatic headaches (PTH). Insights from genomic studies are beginning to unravel how certain genetic markers might influence an individual's response to brain injuries and their subsequent development of headaches.[91] Understanding these genetic factors not only aids in identifying individuals at

higher risk but also paves the way for personalized treatment approaches tailored to an individual's genetic profile..

Personalized Treatment Approaches
With the identification of specific genetic markers associated with PTH, personalized treatment strategies are being developed. These approaches consider an individual's genetic makeup to optimize therapeutic interventions, potentially improving outcomes and reducing the frequency and intensity of headaches following brain injuries, including TBI, mTBI and concussions. This personalized approach can significantly enhance the quality of life for survivors by addressing their unique genetic susceptibilities and needs.

Summary:

- Genetic markers can predict susceptibility to PTH.

- Personalized treatments based on genetics are being developed.

Lifestyle Factors

Sleep Quality and Headache Frequency
Researchers are also delving into the role of lifestyle factors in exacerbating or alleviating post-traumatic headaches. Sleep, nutrition, and stress management, covered extensively in other chapters, are areas where recent studies suggest interventions can make a significant difference. For example, Hou et al. [92] demonstrated that improving sleep hygiene can substantially reduce headache frequency and severity in TBI and mTBI survivors. Addressing sleep disturbances not only alleviates headache symptoms but also enhances overall recovery and quality of life.

Nutrition and Stress Management

Proper nutrition and effective stress management techniques are essential components of comprehensive headache management strategies. Balanced diets rich in essential nutrients support brain health, while stress reduction practices like mindfulness and cognitive-behavioral therapy can mitigate factors that trigger or worsen PTH.

Summary:
- Sleep hygiene significantly impacts headache management..

- Nutrition and stress management are critical for reducing PTH.

Hormonal Influences

Cortisol and Stress-Related Hormones
Brain injuries often disrupt hormonal balances, particularly cortisol and stress-related hormones, which can exacerbate headaches. Understanding these hormonal shifts provides potential pathways for new therapeutic strategies. Research examining hormonal regulation and neuroendocrine dysfunction suggests potential pathways for targeted headache management strategies.[93]

Summary:
- Hormonal imbalances contribute to PTH and chronic migraines.

- Hormonal therapies are being explored as potential treatments.

Technological Innovations

Artificial Intelligence in Headache Management
A notable shift in recent research is the incorporation of technology and artificial intelligence (AI) in the study and treatment of post-traumatic headaches (PTH). AI tools are improving diagnostic accuracy, predicting headache patterns, and personalizing treatment plans for brain injury survivors, including those recovering from TBI, mTBI, concussion, or CTE. By analyzing vast amounts of patient data, these technologies aid in identifying patterns that might not be apparent through traditional methods, thus helping in tailoring individualized care plans.

Summary:
- AI enhances diagnostic and treatment precision for PTH.

- Predictive analytics facilitate personalized headache management.

Alternative and Complementary Therapies

Acupuncture and Mindfulness Meditation
Furthermore, the exploration of alternative and complementary therapies is gaining traction. Treatments such as acupuncture, mindfulness meditation, and biofeedback have shown promise in small-scale studies, leading to larger investigations intended to validate these findings. Their integration into broader treatment plans offers additional avenues for PTH management.

Biofeedback Techniques
The integrative approach aims to address the multifactorial nature of headaches post-brain injury, recognizing that a one-size-fits-all solution is unlikely to be effective for all patients.

Summary:
- Alternative therapies offer additional avenues for PTH management.

- Integrative approaches address the complex nature of post-injury headaches.

Gut-Brain Axis

Role of Gut Microbiota in Headaches
The gut-brain axis is an emerging area of interest, with studies suggesting that gut microbiota influences neuroinflammatory and neurotransmitter pathways. Probiotics have shown promise in managing chronic migraines and may offer new treatment avenues for post-traumatic headaches (PTH).[94] These findings underscore the importance of a holistic approach to headache management, considering the interdependence between various bodily systems.

Summary:

- Gut microbiota impacts neuroinflammatory and neurotransmitter pathways.

- Probiotics may offer new treatment avenues for managing chronic migraines and PTH.

Section Conclusion

Research into headaches resulting from brain injuries, including mTBI, TBI, and CTE, is advancing rapidly. By integrating insights from neurobiology, genetics, lifestyle, and technology, health professionals and caregivers can better manage this debilitating condition. Staying informed of these developments is essential for optimizing care and improving outcomes for survivors.

Chapter 5:
Tracking Headache Patterns

After a brain injury, such as TBI, concussion, or mild traumatic brain injury (mTBI), understanding headache patterns is crucial for effective management. Keeping a headache diary allows individuals to document frequency, intensity, and potential triggers—a practice that reveals vital patterns over time. This habitual tracking helps survivors and caregivers understand behavioral or environmental factors that may exacerbate headache symptoms. Once these patterns emerge, they can significantly inform treatment decisions, allowing healthcare providers to tailor interventions more effectively.[95] Additionally, advancements in technology have introduced several apps, such as Migraine Buddy or Headache Tracker, designed to assist in headache tracking, making it more accessible and thorough.[96] By aligning documented patterns with medical guidance, survivors can develop personalized strategies to alleviate headache distress, ultimately improving their quality of life.

Keeping a Headache Diary: Tracking Frequency, Intensity, and Triggers

Tracking your headache patterns through a headache diary is more than a simple exercise; it's a critical tool for managing life post-brain injury. For many survivors of brain injuries, including TBI, concussion, mTBI, and CTE, the experience of headaches is a frequent, sometimes debilitating reality. Understanding the relationship between the events of daily life and headaches can be instrumental in alleviating some of the burdens they impose.

The process of keeping a headache diary involves documenting the frequency, intensity, and potential triggers of each headache episode. Focus on capturing key details, such as symptoms and any relevant activities or emotions leading to headaches. You don't need to be well-versed in medical jargon to maintain this diary. Instead, focus on capturing key details that can help you and your healthcare provider decipher patterns over time. In a practical sense, this might mean jotting down notes on your headache symptoms and any relevant activities or emotions you experienced in the hours leading up to it.

Frequency measurement is vital because it gives you and your healthcare providers a clearer view of how often these headaches occur. For instance, changes in frequency might correlate with adjustments in medication, stress levels, or sleep patterns.[97]

When it comes to intensity, subjective interpretation plays a role. Rating your headaches on a scale from one to ten can identify patterns related to specific triggers or events. Observing a drop in intensity after certain lifestyle adjustments can signal that you're on the right track in your management approach.

Identifying triggers can be one of the most rewarding aspects of keeping a headache diary. Triggers can be as varied as stress, dietary choices, lack of sleep, dehydration, or sensory sensitivities like bright lights or loud noises, which are common among brain injury survivors.[98] By systematically recording each headache episode's context, you might realize, for instance, that skipping meals leads to increased headache frequency or that exercise reduces symptom severity.

Aside from these core components, a headache diary can include additional factors such as concurrent symptoms, emotional state, and any interventions you attempted, like medication or rest. Over time, this comprehensive record can help you and your healthcare provider fine-tune your treatment regimen.

While traditional pen-and-paper diaries are entirely sufficient and can be gratifyingly tactile, various digital tools and apps can enhance the convenience and depth of your tracking efforts.

Numerous smartphone applications are designed to streamline this process, often offering features like customizable entry forms, reminders, and the ability to easily share the data with healthcare providers. These tools can automatically correlate weather data or even suggest probable triggers based on your inputs.[99]

Despite the logistical benefits, committing to a headache diary can be emotionally taxing. Reliving or anticipating the pain through documentation can feel disheartening at times. It's crucial to approach the diary as a means of empowerment, a way to regain control over a part of life that often feels uncontrollable. Understanding the specific elements that exacerbate or alleviate your headaches puts you back in the driver's seat, offering an initiative-taking strategy to manage your well-being.

The data collected through your headache diary can also be instrumental during medical consultations. Rather than relying on memory, which can be fallible during stressful episodes, you can present your healthcare provider with concrete evidence for review and consideration. This clarity not only facilitates more accurate diagnoses but can also encourage more personalized, effective treatment plans that are responsive to your unique needs.

Furthermore, involving caregivers in this process can enhance support systems, providing additional perspectives that might be overlooked or forgotten. Caregivers can help ensure consistent diary maintenance, offer insights from an outside viewpoint, and engage more meaningfully with your journey to recovery.

A headache diary isn't just a record; it's a powerful instrument for change. It's about taking incremental steps to understand and improve your quality of life. By diligently tracking your headache patterns, you're setting the stage for effective intervention and ultimately, a more comfortable existence post-injury. Take the time to document, review, and adapt—because each entry brings you closer to understanding yourself, your triggers, and your paths to relief.

Using Patterns to Inform Treatment Choices

Tracking headache patterns through consistent observation and documentation is a cornerstone in effectively managing post-traumatic headaches (PTH) following a brain injury. Once these patterns are identified, they can directly inform treatment choices tailored to each individual's unique circumstances. Post-traumatic headaches in brain injury survivors, including those with TBI, mTBI, and concussion, are complex, often blending features from tension-type, migraine, and cluster headaches, making a one-size-fits-all approach ineffective. Instead, a personalized treatment plan guided by documented patterns offers the most potential for relief.

Recognizing patterns in headache frequency, intensity, and triggers is essential for shaping treatment strategies. For brain injury survivors, understanding the nuances of their post-injury headaches can highlight specific triggers such as light sensitivity, overstimulation, or cognitive overload. By keeping a headache diary, survivors can document these patterns over time, enabling healthcare providers to create individualized plans that incorporate both medical and lifestyle interventions.[100]

Survivors of TBI, mTBI, and concussion often experience heightened sensitivity to stimuli—such as bright lights, loud noises, or chaotic environments—that can significantly influence headache patterns. Studies show that light sensitivity (photophobia) and sound sensitivity (phonophobia) exacerbate headache symptoms across brain injuries.[101] Recognizing these triggers allows for tailored interventions, such as using tinted glasses, noise-canceling headphones, or practicing gradual desensitization techniques.

Additionally, headaches resulting from brain injuries may stem from disrupted nociceptive pathways and neuroinflammation, requiring targeted pharmacological and non-pharmacological treatments. For example, medications that address neurogenic inflammation, such as CGRP inhibitors, have shown promise in alleviating persistent headaches in post-traumatic cases.[102].

Healthcare Provider Involvement

Communication with healthcare providers is critical when managing post-traumatic headaches. Sharing headache diaries and patterns with neurologists or rehabilitation specialists ensures that all aspects of an individual's condition are considered. Providers may adjust medication regimens, suggest physical or cognitive therapies, or recommend biofeedback and mindfulness practices as part of a holistic approach.

Example:
In cases where stress and anxiety amplify headaches, cognitive-behavioral therapy (CBT) has been effective in helping brain injury survivors, including those with TBI, mTBI, or concussion, manage emotional triggers and reduce headache frequency.[103]

Emphasizing Technology's Role

Technology offers valuable support in tracking and analyzing headache patterns. Apps designed for headache monitoring, such as Migraine Buddy, Headache Log, or N1-Headache, can simplify this process, often providing insights that might not be apparent through manual tracking. These tools can assist in correlating headaches with environmental factors, dietary habits, or behavior changes, offering a clearer picture of potential triggers and influences.[104]

Recommendations for Caregivers and Survivors

Caregivers play a vital role in supporting brain injury survivors by assisting with consistent tracking and offering insights that individuals might overlook. By fostering open communication and engaging in shared monitoring efforts, caregivers contribute to a collaborative recovery process.

Lifestyle Modifications

In addition to medication adjustments, lifestyle modifications can play a significant role in headache management. For instance, if a headache diary indicates that physical exertion exacerbates symptoms, a gradual and supervised increase in physical activity might be advised. This progressive approach can help build endurance while reducing the likelihood of triggering a headache. Patterns revealed through tracking enable healthcare providers to make adjustments that maximize therapeutic benefits while minimizing adverse effects.[97]

Diet and Nutrition

Diet and nutrition are equally critical aspects of using patterns to inform treatment choices. Identifying foods or additives that consistently trigger headaches can lead to dietary changes that reduce headache frequency. For example, if a preserved meat product consistently correlates with headache onset, eliminating it from the diet may help. Establishing a record of correlations empowers individuals and their healthcare providers to make informed dietary adjustments. [97][98]

Sleep Patterns

Diet and nutrition are equally critical aspects of using patterns to inform treatment choices. Identifying foods or additives that consistently trigger headaches can lead to dietary changes that reduce headache frequency. For example, if a preserved meat product consistently correlates with headache onset, eliminating it from the diet may help. Establishing a record of correlations empowers individuals and their healthcare providers to make informed dietary adjustments.

Communication with Healthcare Providers

Communicating identified patterns to healthcare providers enables a collaborative approach to treatment. This communication helps ensure that all aspects of an individual's lifestyle and medical history are considered when crafting a personalized treatment plan. Regular follow-ups are important for evaluating the effectiveness of the chosen strategies, making necessary adjustments based on ongoing pattern observations.

Adapting Management Strategies

The dynamic and often interconnected nature of headache patterns requires flexibility in management strategies. Treatment plans should be regularly revisited and updated to reflect new insights gained from continuous pattern tracking. This adaptable approach helps maximize the effectiveness of headache management, improving outcomes for those living with post-traumatic headaches.[95]

Empowering Survivors and Caregivers

Ultimately, leveraging patterns to inform treatment confirms the importance of a patient-centered approach. Each headache experience is unique, shaped by a complex interplay of biological, psychological, and environmental factors. Understanding these individual differences through diligent pattern tracking and analysis empowers survivors and their caregivers. With growing knowledge about specific triggers and effective interventions, the potential to enhance quality of life and reduce the burden of post-traumatic headaches becomes increasingly attainable.[105]

Refining Treatment Through Pattern Recognition

Recognizing and understanding headache patterns play a crucial role in informing effective treatment choices for brain injury survivors. This individualized approach guides medical and lifestyle interventions and empowers individuals to take an active role in managing their condition.

By continually adapting to insights on headache patterns, survivors and their healthcare providers can work collaboratively to refine strategies, achieving better symptom control and an improved quality of life. The ability to track and respond to patterns ensures that care remains flexible and responsive, addressing the unique challenges faced by everyone.

Tracking Headache Patterns Tools and Apps for Monitoring Headaches

Harnessing Technology for Headache Management
In the ever-evolving landscape of digital health, tools and apps have become invaluable companions for managing headaches after brain injuries. While traditional methods like pen-and-paper headache diaries remain effective, the integration of technology offers several advantages, including ease of use, data analysis capabilities, and real-time tracking. These digital solutions can help survivors of TBI, mTBI, concussion, and CTE, along with their caregivers, gain a clearer understanding of pain patterns, triggers, and ultimately improve headache management.[106]

Comprehensive Data Collection and Integration
One of the primary benefits of headache apps is their ability to record comprehensive data sets effortlessly. These tools allow users to input details such as headache intensity, duration, and possible triggers. Many apps also integrate with wearable devices, automatically tracking physiological parameters like sleep patterns and physical activity levels.[107] This integration offers a holistic view of the factors contributing to headache occurrences and can guide more precise intervention strategies.

Identifying Patterns and Triggers
Apps often include features that help identify headache patterns over time. This is particularly useful for survivors dealing with post-traumatic headaches, as it helps discern the unique combination of triggers, such as light sensitivity, stress levels, or dietary factors.[107] Recognizing these triggers allows users to make informed adjustments, including lifestyle changes or medical interventions, to reduce headache frequency and severity.

Facilitating Communication with Healthcare Providers
Data collected through headache apps can greatly enhance communication with healthcare providers. Survivors often struggle to accurately recount their headache history due to memory lapses

or cognitive fatigue, challenges commonly faced by brain injury survivors. Digital records provide organized and precise data that healthcare professionals can analyze, improving diagnosis accuracy and supporting the development of personalized treatment plans.

Noteworthy Headache Apps
Several apps designed specifically for headache and migraine monitoring stand out:

MigraineBuddy: Acclaimed for its user-friendly interface, comprehensive tracking features, and community support aspect.

Headache Log: Focuses on simple tracking with minimal input, ideal for those experiencing severe symptoms.

N1-Headache: Specializes in customized data collection and analysis, generating individualized insights for crafting tailored coping strategies.[107] These tools are useful for all survivors of brain injuries, offering flexibility to adapt to their unique needs and preferences

Consistency in Use and Limitations

For all brain injury survivors, adherence to a consistent documentation routine is key to maximizing the effectiveness of headache tracking tools. Regular entries enable users to monitor treatment efficacy and make timely adjustments, ultimately contributing to an improved quality of life. Survivors and caregivers should collaborate with healthcare providers to select apps that align with their specific needs. However, it's essential to remember that these tools should complement—not replace—professional guidance, ensuring that any technology use aligns with a broader, supervised medical strategy.[106]

Empowering Brain Injury Survivors
The intersection of technology and headache management represents an exciting frontier for survivors of TBI, mTBI, concussion, and CTE. These tools empower individuals to take an active role in their recovery, enabling better self-awareness and

control over their condition. As digital health technologies continue to advance, future developments promise even more individualized insights and interventions, helping survivors better navigate their recovery journey.[107]

Chapter 6:
The Role of Sleep in Headache Management

Sleep plays a pivotal role in managing headaches, especially for those coping with a traumatic brain injury (TBI), mild traumatic brain injury (mTBI), concussion, or chronic traumatic encephalopathy (CTE). Research suggests that poor sleep quality can increase both the severity and frequency of headaches.[108] This relationship is particularly critical for brain injury survivors, including mTBI patients, who often face unique sleep disturbances such as insomnia, fragmented sleep, or hypersomnia. These sleep challenges can significantly exacerbate headache symptoms and delay recovery.

Disrupted sleep patterns are among the most persistent and under-recognized symptoms following brain injury. Even seemingly minor injuries can interfere with the brain's natural sleep-wake cycle, leading to fatigue, cognitive fog, and increased headache susceptibility. Developing a brain-healthy sleep routine is instrumental in breaking this vicious cycle. Prioritizing consistent sleep schedules, creating a restful environment, and addressing underlying sleep disorders like insomnia or sleep apnea may lead to noticeable improvements.[109]

Alongside these changes, practical strategies—such as reducing screen time before bed, avoiding caffeine in the afternoon, and incorporating relaxation techniques—can foster better sleep.[110] Small adjustments, like using earplugs, blackout curtains, or white noise machines, can also make a meaningful difference in improving sleep quality and, subsequently, headache frequency for survivors of brain injuries.

Acknowledging sleep's significant impact empowers survivors of TBI, mTBI, concussion, and CTE to take active steps toward better headache management and overall well-being. With improved sleep hygiene and targeted interventions, survivors can experience reduced headache frequency, improved cognitive function, and an enhanced quality of life.

How Sleep Impacts Headache Severity and Frequency

Sleep is an essential component of brain health, and its role in managing headache severity and frequency in individuals who have suffered a traumatic brain injury (TBI), mild traumatic brain injury (mTBI), concussion, or Chronic Traumatic Encephalopathy (CTE) cannot be overstated. These conditions often disrupt normal sleep patterns, leading to a cycle of sleep deprivation and worsening headaches. For survivors and their caregivers, understanding the intricate connection between sleep and headaches can be crucial in managing symptoms and improving quality of life.

Research has consistently shown that poor sleep exacerbates headaches, both by increasing their frequency and intensity.[111] Disrupted sleep cycles, including insomnia, sleep apnea, and Restless Legs Syndrome (RLS), are common after brain injuries and are strongly associated with more severe post-traumatic headaches.[111] Addressing these sleep disturbances can significantly reduce headache frequency, making sleep management an integral part of headache treatment.

But why does insufficient sleep lead to more severe headaches? One explanation lies in the way sleep affects the body's pain-processing systems. Sleep deprivation can lower the pain threshold and alter the perception of pain.[112] These effects are often heightened in individuals with brain injuries, where even minor sleep disruptions can amplify headache pain. During restful sleep, the body undergoes numerous restorative processes, including the regulation of pain pathways. Disruptions in these processes can intensify sensitivity to pain, making headaches more severe.

Moreover, the relationship between sleep and headaches is bidirectional. Poor sleep can lead to headaches, while persistent headaches can interfere with achieving restorative sleep, creating a vicious cycle that is hard to break. Survivors may find themselves trapped in a pattern where sleep deprivation fuels headaches, and headaches prevent them from sleeping well. Breaking this cycle through better sleep management is a critical step toward recovery.

One key factor to consider is the role of circadian rhythms. Our bodies follow a natural daily cycle, and disruptions to this rhythm can lead to sleep disturbances, which, in turn, affect headache patterns. Factors like staying up too late, irregular sleep schedules, and excessive exposure to artificial light can disturb these rhythms, increasing headache frequency.[113] Maintaining a consistent sleep schedule, limiting screen time before bed, and ensuring a dark sleeping environment can help regulate these rhythms and may consequently reduce headaches.

For caregivers and health professionals working with brain injury survivors, fostering an environment that promotes healthy sleep can make a significant difference in headache management. Creating a brain-friendly sleep routine that prioritizes quality over quantity is essential. This involves not just addressing sleep duration but also focusing on sleep quality.

Adopting good sleep hygiene practices can also empower survivors to better manage their headaches. These practices include setting consistent sleep and wake times, creating a calming pre-sleep routine, and addressing potential sleep disorders with medical guidance. Avoiding caffeine and heavy meals before bedtime and engaging in regular physical activity can further improve sleep quality.

The emotional and psychological impacts of poor sleep also warrant attention. Anxiety and depression, common after brain injuries, can both contribute to and result from poor sleep patterns. These mood disorders significantly affect how individuals perceive and cope with headaches, creating another pathway through which sleep quality impacts headache severity.[112] Addressing these emotional factors can enhance both sleep and headache management outcomes.

Recognizing and addressing sleep issues offers dual benefits for brain injury survivors: improved sleep can reduce headache symptoms, and reduced headache symptoms can lead to better sleep. Tackling these challenges directly empowers survivors to manage their headaches and enhance their overall well-being.

Future research will undoubtedly shed more light on the complex relationship between sleep and headache mechanisms in TBI, mTBI, and concussion survivors, paving the way for more targeted interventions. In the meantime, integrating sleep management into headache treatment plans remains a practical and powerful strategy for overcoming these debilitating symptoms.

Creating a Brain-Friendly Sleep Environment

Headaches caused by brain injuries can be both frustrating and debilitating. A critical aspect of managing these headaches is fostering a sleep routine that supports brain health. While earlier sections explored the relationship between sleep and headaches, this section focuses on practical implementation strategies for creating a sleep-friendly environment.

1. Establish a Consistent Sleep Schedule
A consistent sleep schedule is vital for regulating the body's internal clock. Aim to wake up and go to bed at the same time daily, even on weekends. This stability reduces disruptions that can exacerbate headaches and supports cognitive recovery.[114]

2. Develop a Calming Pre-Sleep Routine
Signal to your brain and body that it's time to wind down with relaxing activities like:

- Reading a book.

- Practicing deep breathing or meditation.

- Gentle yoga stretches.

- Avoid screens at least an hour before sleep, as blue light disrupts melatonin production.[115]

3. Optimize the Sleep Environment

Create a bedroom that promotes restful sleep:

- Keep the room cool, quiet, and dark.

- Use **white noise machines**, **earplugs**, or **light-blocking curtains** to minimize disruptions.

- Invest in comfortable, supportive bedding to reduce physical strain.

4. Mindfulness and Stress Reduction

Incorporating mindfulness practices into your bedtime routine can reduce stress and anxiety, common hurdles for brain injury survivors. Techniques such as meditation, body scanning, or journaling can calm the mind, helping to process thoughts and create mental space for relaxation. This approach is particularly beneficial for survivors who often experience heightened anxiety or mental fatigue.[116]

5. Dietary and Lifestyle Adjustments

Diet and Nutrition

Caffeine, nicotine, and alcohol can disrupt sleep when consumed late in the day. Adjusting the timing of these substances, or reducing their intake altogether, can significantly improve sleep quality. Avoiding heavy meals late in the evening also helps ensure uninterrupted sleep, allowing the body to recover effectively.[117]

Physical Activity and Sleep

Physical activity supports the establishment of a healthy sleep cycle. Regular exercise reduces stress, improves mood, and promotes better sleep. However, timing is crucial: strenuous workouts close to bedtime can leave you feeling alert rather than relaxed. Instead, aim to exercise earlier in the day to foster both physical well-being and improved sleep.[118]

Developing a Balanced Routine

Balancing these factors—diet, physical activity, and sleep routines—forms the foundation for a brain-friendly lifestyle. Making small but consistent adjustments can have a cumulative positive effect on sleep quality and headache management.[117]

6. Seek Professional Guidance

Persistent sleep disturbances may require professional intervention. Cognitive-behavioral therapy for insomnia (CBT-I) and sleep studies can uncover underlying issues, such as **sleep apnea**, that require targeted treatments.[119]

Practical Strategies for Better Sleep

To consolidate the strategies outlined in this chapter:

- **Be consistent:** Maintain regular sleep and wake times.

- **Create the right environment:** Minimize light, noise, and discomfort.

- **Use tools:** Journals and apps can help track sleep patterns.

- **Work with professionals:** Seek specialized care for persistent issues.

Next Steps in Sleep and Headache Management

This Key Points Review serves as a practical summary of the sleep strategies discussed in this chapter. By implementing even a few of these practices, survivors and caregivers can make meaningful progress toward improving sleep quality, reducing headache frequency, and enhancing overall well-being. For brain injury survivors, including those recovering from TBI, mTBI, concussion, or CTE, patience and persistence are essential, as improvements in sleep patterns often require time, consistency, and small, sustainable adjustments to fully stabilize.

Remember, overcoming sleep challenges is a journey, but with dedication and support, the rewards can be transformative.

Resources and Guidance for Better Sleep and Headache Management

Managing sleep disturbances and headaches after brain injuries, including TBI, mTBI, concussion, and CTE, often requires a mix of self-help strategies and professional guidance. Below are actionable resources, professional recommendations, and further reading to assist survivors and caregivers.

When to Consult Professionals

Certain sleep and headache challenges require specialized care. Persistent issues should prompt consultation with professionals familiar with brain injury rehabilitation, such as:

- **Sleep Specialists:** For insomnia, sleep apnea, or other unexplained sleep disturbances that worsen headaches. Many clinics offer sliding-scale fees or accept Medicare/Medicaid.

- **Neurologists:** For chronic headaches resistant to sleep management strategies or accompanied by neurological symptoms like confusion or weakness.

- **Cognitive Behavioral Therapists (CBT-I Specialists):** To address sleep disorders through Cognitive Behavioral Therapy for Insomnia (CBT-I), proven effective for brain injury survivors.

- **Occupational Therapists:** To assist in creating routines and modifying environments that promote better sleep and reduce headache triggers.

- **Support Groups and Peer Networks:** Online and in-person groups for brain injury survivors provide emotional support and practical advice. Sharing experiences helps build resilience and discover effective coping strategies.

Affordable Resources for Sleep and Headache Care

For individuals on limited income, consider the following options:

- **Community Health Clinics**: Many offer free or low-cost sleep studies or headache management programs.

- **Local Libraries**: Access to books on sleep hygiene, mindfulness, and brain health.

- **Apps and Online Tools**: Many free apps, such as Insight Timer for meditation or MigraineBuddy for headache tracking, can be helpful.

Recommended Readings and Tools

Explore these resources for deeper insights into sleep and headache management:

1. **"Cognitive Behavioral Treatment for Sleep Disorders in the Primary Care Setting" by Rains et al., 2015**

   o A deep dive into CBT techniques for managing sleep disorders and their role in reducing headache symptoms.

2. **"Sleep and Headaches: A Common Association with Important Clinical Implications" by Rains, 2018**

   o Explores the bidirectional relationship between sleep disturbances and headaches.

3. **"Mindfulness Meditation and Sleep Quality Among Older Adults" by Black et al., 2015**

   o Discusses how mindfulness practices can improve sleep and overall well-being.

4. **"The Association of Sleep and Pain" by Finan et al., 2013**

   o Examines how sleep quality impacts pain perception, particularly in individuals with chronic headaches.

5. **"Evening Use of Light-Emitting Devices and Circadian Disruption" by Chang et al., 2015**

- o Details how screen time affects sleep quality and provides actionable advice for reducing its impact.

Empowering Sustainable Change

Addressing sleep disturbances can significantly improve headache management and quality of life. Building small, consistent habits—like maintaining a sleep schedule and creating a restful environment—helps survivors take control of their recovery. With time and dedication, these efforts lead to meaningful, lasting improvements for TBI, mTBI, concussion, and CTE survivors.

Chapter 7:
Nutrition for Headache Relief

Nutrition is a cornerstone of headache management for survivors of TBI, mTBI, concussion, and CTE. The foods we eat influence inflammation, pain pathways, and even neurological recovery, making dietary choices an essential part of a comprehensive treatment plan. Anti-inflammatory foods, such as leafy greens, fatty fish, and nuts, can reduce headache frequency and intensity by calming overactive pain pathways.[120] Conversely, certain foods, like processed meats or artificial sweeteners, may act as triggers, intensifying headache symptoms.

Hydration is another key element, as even mild dehydration can exacerbate headache pain by affecting blood flow and neural signaling.[121] Additionally, supplements like magnesium, riboflavin, and omega-3 fatty acids offer targeted benefits, helping survivors address deficiencies that may worsen symptoms.[122]

By understanding how food, hydration, and supplements interact with the brain's recovery process, survivors, caregivers, and healthcare providers can make informed dietary choices. This chapter explores the science behind these nutritional strategies, offering practical guidance for improving headache management and enhancing quality of life.

Balancing Nutrition for Headache Relief

Nutrition significantly influences headache frequency, intensity, and duration in survivors of brain injuries like TBI, mTBI, concussion, and CTE. A balanced approach involves incorporating foods and nutrients that reduce inflammation while avoiding those that act as triggers.

Nutrients and Foods That Help

Omega-3 Fatty Acids

Omega 3 fatty acids, found in fatty fish like salmon, mackerel, and sardines, omega-3s have anti-inflammatory properties and may reduce headache severity, especially in chronic cases.[123] For plant-based options, include flaxseeds or walnuts in your diet.

Magnesium-Rich Foods

Studies suggest low magnesium levels are associated with more frequent headaches.[124] Incorporate spinach, pumpkin seeds, and almonds, which are versatile and easy to include in meals.

Riboflavin (Vitamin B2)

Riboflavin supports mitochondrial energy production, which may reduce headache frequency.[125] Good sources include eggs, lean meats, and milk.

Hydrating Foods

Dehydration is a well-known trigger for headaches.[126] While water is essential, hydrating foods like cucumbers, watermelons, and oranges can boost your fluid intake.

Foods That May Worsen Headaches

Processed Meats

Preservatives like nitrates or nitrites in deli meats, sausages, and bacon may trigger headaches by dilating blood vessels.[127] Consider nitrate-free alternatives.

Artificial Sweeteners

Aspartame and other artificial sweeteners have been linked to headaches in some individuals. While evidence is limited, it may help to reduce or eliminate these from your diet.[128]

Histamine-Rich Foods
Aged cheeses, fermented products, and certain alcoholic drinks (e.g., red wine) can affect histamine metabolism, potentially triggering headaches.[129]

Alcohol
Alcohol acts as a diuretic and disrupts sleep, compounding issues for those with post-traumatic headaches. Consider limiting or avoiding it.

Caffeine
Small amounts of caffeine may relieve headaches by constricting blood vessels. However, irregular intake, overconsumption, or withdrawal can be triggers.[130] Balance is key.

Actionable Takeaways

- Keep a food diary to track potential triggers.

- Focus on anti-inflammatory foods like leafy greens and fatty fish.

- Limit or avoid processed meats, excess caffeine, and alcohol.

The Role of Hydration in Headache Prevention

Hydration is a fundamental yet often overlooked aspect of headache management. The brain, composed of approximately 70% water, relies on adequate fluid levels to function properly. Dehydration can shrink brain tissues, trigger pain receptors, and exacerbate headaches.[121] This issue is particularly relevant for brain injury survivors, where fluid balance is critical in minimizing inflammation and promoting recovery.

Physiological Impacts of Dehydration:
Reduced Blood Flow: Dehydration lowers blood volume, which hampers oxygen and nutrient delivery to the brain, potentially worsening headaches.[131]

Electrolyte Imbalance:
Sodium and potassium disruptions can lead to increased neural firing and muscle tension, creating a fertile ground for headaches.[132]

Recognizing symptoms of dehydration is the first step in prevention and management. These symptoms might include dry mouth, fatigue, dizziness, a decrease in urine output, and of course, headache. When individuals have cognitive impairments due to their brain injury, caregivers play a critical role in regularly monitoring and encouraging fluid intake.

Habitual hydration practices can be introduced into daily routines. Drinking water regularly throughout the day rather than in large amounts at once helps maintain optimal hydration levels. This is crucial for headache management. It prevents the peaks and troughs in fluid levels that can inadvertently trigger headaches. Implementing reminders or setting alarm cues can be beneficial, particularly for individuals with memory issues stemming from their brain injury.

The source of hydration is equally important to consider. While water is the purest form of hydration, beverages such as herbal teas and electrolyte-infused drinks can also be beneficial. Care should be taken to avoid excessive intake of caffeinated and sugary drinks, which can contribute to dehydration and possibly provoke headaches.[133] A balanced approach, with guidance from healthcare providers, can help tailor fluid intake according to individual needs and preferences.

Moreover, food choices contribute significantly to daily hydration. Many fruits and vegetables, such as cucumbers, strawberries, and watermelon, have high water content and provide vitamins and minerals crucial for brain recovery. Including these in the diet helps reinforce hydration efforts and offers an enjoyable way to ensure fluid intake without relying solely on beverages.

Understanding personal hydration needs involves acknowledging factors such as body size, local climate, and activity level. Individuals recovering from brain injuries might have varying requirements based on these factors, coupled with their stage of recovery and any additional medical conditions. Consulting healthcare practitioners can offer personalized recommendations, ensuring hydration strategies are effectively incorporated into broader headache management plans.

While improving hydration alone may not completely eradicate headaches, it represents a significant, manageable component of a holistic headache management plan. It is a foundational practice that supports other interventions such as nutrition, sleep, stress management, and medication. The simplicity of maintaining proper hydration offers a practical, low-cost intervention that can empower individuals and caregivers alike, giving them an attainable tactic in the fight against headaches.

The road to managing headaches for TBI, concussion, and CTE survivors is complex and multifaceted. However, focusing on hydration can lead to tangible improvements, reducing headache frequency and intensity while supporting the injured brain's overall recovery and well-being. With consistent hydration practices in place, survivors can experience fewer obstacles in their healing journey, leading to improved quality of life and enhanced day-to-day functioning.

Research-Backed Nutritional Strategies and Supplements

For individuals recovering from traumatic brain injuries (TBI), including mild traumatic brain injury (mTBI), concussions, or chronic traumatic encephalopathy (CTE), headaches often present a significant roadblock to improving quality of life. While many remedies may be considered, nutritional strategies stand out for their ability to provide relief naturally and support overall health. Recent research has shed light on how targeted dietary choices and supplements can significantly contribute to headache management, offering a foundation for strategies that can be adapted to personal needs.

First and foremost, maintaining a balanced diet rich in specific nutrients can act as a cornerstone for alleviating headaches. Magnesium, a mineral that's crucial for numerous biological processes, has shown potential in reducing the frequency and intensity of migraines and other headache types. It plays a role in preventing the excessive excitation of neurons, a contributor to headaches and migraines. Foods like leafy greens, nuts, and whole grains are excellent sources of magnesium and can be easily incorporated into meals.[134]

In addition to magnesium, riboflavin, or vitamin B2, is gaining recognition in scientific circles for its promise in headache prevention. It's believed that riboflavin enhances mitochondrial function, making energy production in brain cells more efficient and, consequently, reducing the likelihood of headaches. Studies suggest that a dosage of 400 mg of riboflavin daily can lower migraine frequency; hence, enriching one's diet with foods such as eggs, dairy products, and almonds, or considering supplements, might prove beneficial.[135]

Another critical nutrient is omega-3 fatty acids, primarily found in fish like salmon and sardines as well as in flaxseeds and walnuts. These polyunsaturated fats have anti-inflammatory properties, which can be crucial in mitigating headache symptoms associated with inflammation—a common issue in post-traumatic headache scenarios. Some research indicates that a diet high in omega-3s could reduce headache severity and frequency, providing a more dietary approach to pain management.[136]

Hydration cannot be overlooked when discussing nutritional strategies for headache relief. Dehydration is a well-known trigger for headaches. Ensuring adequate fluid intake, preferably through water, herbal teas, and hydrating fruits and vegetables, can be a simple yet powerful strategy to mitigate headaches. In cases where maintaining hydration poses a challenge, monitoring daily intake and setting reminders might assist in forming a consistent habit that supports headache management.

Let's not forget about the importance of avoiding specific dietary triggers. While individual triggers can vary, some culprits commonly worsen headaches. These include alcohol, particularly red wine, aged cheeses, and foods containing monosodium glutamate (MSG) or preservatives. Through dietary tracking and patience, individuals can better identify and then steer clear of these triggers, potentially reducing headache occurrences.

Beyond individual nutrients, comprehensive diets like the Mediterranean diet have been lauded for their overall health benefits and potentially minimizing headaches. This diet emphasizes fruits, vegetables, whole grains, fish, and healthy fats (mainly from olive oil), creating a balanced approach that is not only heart-healthy but potentially headache-fighting. The intricate balance of anti-inflammatory and antioxidant-rich foods offers a holistic approach to wellness which may also reflect positively in headache management.

Turning to supplements, Coenzyme Q10, a naturally occurring antioxidant, has been identified as a valuable ally in headache relief. It supports mitochondrial function, similar to riboflavin, providing cells with the energy required for proper functioning. Research suggests that daily supplementation of CoQ10 may reduce the number of days headaches occur, thus signaling another potential component of headache management.[137]

In terms of practical application, seeking the guidance of healthcare professionals when incorporating supplements is recommended. Not only will they ensure that these supplements won't interfere with any other medications, but they can also recommend appropriate dosages, tailoring plans to suit individual health needs and goals.

Conclusively, navigating headache relief through nutritional strategies demands an integrated approach that considers both dietary inclusions and exclusions, hydration, and supplementation. Undertaking these strategies, TBI, mTBI, concussion, and CTE survivors might find themselves better equipped to manage headaches effectively, bolstering their progress toward recovery and enhanced quality of life.

While research continues to evolve, these nutritional strategies offer promising routes to alleviate headaches for those affected by brain injuries. By adopting these methods, there is hope for reducing headache frequency and intensity, ultimately leading to a more manageable recovery process.

Chapter 8:
Stress Management Techniques

In the journey of managing post-traumatic headaches, understanding and reducing stress plays a pivotal role. Traumatic brain injury (TBI), mild traumatic brain injury (mTBI), concussion, and chronic traumatic encephalopathy (CTE) can intensify stress responses, exacerbating headache symptoms.[138] Integrating stress management techniques such as mindfulness, meditation, and relaxation exercises can aid in alleviating headache frequency and severity, providing a path towards improved well-being.

Practicing mindfulness, for instance, enhances present-moment awareness, which can diminish stress responses and lead to a reduction in headache occurrences.[138] Developing a consistent stress-reduction routine tailored to individual needs not only empowers survivors but also fosters resilience against triggering headaches. Techniques such as guided imagery or controlled breathing have been shown to contribute to a more balanced stress response, which is essential for managing post-traumatic symptoms effectively.[147] While the strategies may vary for each person, the commitment to addressing stress can catalyze a transformative impact on quality of life.

The Impact of Stress on Post-Traumatic Headaches

Post-traumatic headaches (PTH) are a frequent consequence of traumatic brain injury (TBI), mild traumatic brain injury (mTBI), concussion, and chronic traumatic encephalopathy (CTE). Stress is a noteworthy factor that can exacerbate these headaches, significantly affecting survivors and their caregivers. Understanding the impact of stress on PTH is essential for improving quality of life after a brain injury. Stress management is not just therapeutic—it is essential for managing and potentially reducing the frequency and intensity of these headaches.

Stress triggers a complex set of physiological responses in the body. When subject to stress, the body releases hormones like adrenaline and cortisol, which prepare the body for 'fight or flight' responses. While these reactions are beneficial in short bursts, prolonged stress can lead to increased headache frequency and intensity. For individuals already dealing with PTH, this stress-induced cycle can become a burdensome loop, making stress management critically important.[138]

Moreover, stress can disrupt natural serotonin levels in the brain—a neurotransmitter critical for regulating mood and pain. Fluctuations in serotonin can heighten pain sensitivity, often triggering headaches or migraines that are more intense and resistant to treatment. (Zeidan et al., 2015)[139] For survivors of brain injury, this interplay between stress, serotonin, and pain underscores the importance of actively managing stress to mitigate its physiological and neurological impacts.

Stress also increases muscle tension, particularly around the neck and shoulders, which is a significant trigger for tension-type headaches. In those with a history of brain injury, this muscle tension can exacerbate or transform into severe PTH.[140] Combined with the hormonal and neurochemical effects of stress, these physical responses create a compounding cycle that heightens headache susceptibility.

Additionally, the psychological toll of living with a brain injury inherently introduces stress. Factors such as managing symptoms, adapting to changes in employment, and navigating shifts in personal relationships can contribute to chronic anxiety. This persistent stress not only lowers the threshold for headache activation but also perpetuates a cycle of emotional strain and physical pain, further complicating recovery. (Stocchetti & Zanier, 2016)[141]

Adopting effective stress management techniques can break this vicious cycle. Mindfulness and meditation are powerful tools that help calm the mind and reduce stress. Studies have shown that consistent mindfulness practice can lower cortisol levels and reduce headache frequency.[138] Biofeedback, which trains individuals to regulate physiological processes like heart rate and muscle tension, also shows promise in reducing stress-related headache severity.[142] Progressive muscle relaxation (PMR), involving the systematic tensing and releasing of muscle groups, can further alleviate tension and mitigate stress-induced headaches.[142]

Creating a personalized stress-reduction plan empowers survivors and caregivers alike, giving them more control over their headaches. While eliminating stress entirely is unrealistic, reducing exposure to major stressors and adopting healthier coping mechanisms can make a meaningful difference. Seeking professional support, such as therapy or cognitive-behavioral therapy (CBT), can also provide targeted strategies for managing both stress and headaches .

Summarizing, the connection between stress and post-traumatic headaches underscores the importance of proactive stress management as part of a comprehensive approach to recovery. By addressing stressors through mindfulness, relaxation techniques, and professional support, survivors and their caregivers can improve their resilience and overall quality of life.

Mindfulness, Meditation, and Relaxation Techniques

Stress can be a formidable challenge for anyone, but for those experiencing headaches after a traumatic brain injury (TBI), mild traumatic brain injury (mTBI), concussion, or chronic traumatic encephalopathy (CTE), managing stress effectively is crucial. Implementing mindfulness, meditation, and relaxation techniques offers viable pathways to alleviate the exacerbation of headaches brought on by stress. These practices foster a calm mental state, bringing about physiological changes that can reduce headache frequency and intensity.

Mindfulness involves being present in the moment, paying attention to thoughts, feelings, and bodily sensations without judgment. Research indicates that mindfulness helps modulate the neural pathways associated with stress, making it an effective method for managing post-traumatic headaches.[143] By cultivating an awareness of mental states, mindfulness allows individuals to recognize early signs of stress, thus preventing the escalation of headache symptoms.

For individuals with brain injuries, mindfulness-based stress reduction (MBSR) has been shown to be particularly effective in managing comorbid conditions like chronic insomnia. Studies highlight that MBSR not only improves sleep but also lowers cortisol levels, reducing overall stress. These changes can play a significant role in managing post-traumatic headaches and improving the quality of life for survivors.[144]

Implementing mindfulness doesn't have to be complex. Incorporating simple mindful breathing exercises into a daily routine can be highly beneficial. For instance, spending just a few minutes focusing on inhalation and exhalation throughout the day can lead to reduced stress and a deeper sense of awareness. Over time, such practices can provide cumulative benefits, helping to manage stress more effectively and alleviate headaches.

Meditation, a practice closely related to mindfulness, involves sitting quietly and focusing attention on a specific object, thought, or activity. Regular meditation has been shown to decrease stress hormone levels while increasing the production of serotonin, a neurotransmitter that helps regulate mood and pain. These biochemical effects may offer relief for tension headaches and migraines.[145] Guided meditations, particularly those designed for stress and headache management, are widely available and can be helpful for beginners.

For individuals who are new to meditation, starting with short guided sessions can be a practical way to build confidence. Apps and online resources tailored to stress management provide step-by-step instructions, enabling survivors to gradually integrate meditation into their daily lives.

Relaxation techniques encompass a broader range of practices aimed at promoting physical and mental peace. One effective method is **progressive muscle relaxation (PMR)**, which involves tensing and then slowly releasing specific muscle groups. This practice can reduce the physical tension associated with stress and tension-type headaches.[146] PMR is particularly beneficial for individuals with post-traumatic headaches, as it directly targets the muscle tightness that often accompanies stress.

Another relaxation technique is **guided imagery**, which involves visualizing calming and serene settings. This mental exercise provides a reprieve from the physical and emotional discomfort of headaches while reducing stress responses in the brain. Regularly engaging in guided imagery sessions can foster a sense of calm and emotional balance, further supporting headache management.

Consistency in practicing mindfulness, meditation, and relaxation techniques is key to their effectiveness. Even dedicating a few minutes daily to these practices can yield significant reductions in stress levels and headache intensity over time. For caregivers, participating in these activities alongside survivors can strengthen emotional bonds and create a shared sense of peace.

The scientific backing for mindfulness, meditation, and relaxation techniques continues to grow, underscoring their efficacy in reducing stress-related symptoms, particularly post-traumatic headaches. These non-invasive practices, when integrated into a comprehensive stress management plan, provide survivors with tools to enhance both mental well-being and headache relief.

Developing a Stress-Reduction Routine

Living with a traumatic brain injury, mild traumatic brain injury (mTBI), concussion, or chronic traumatic encephalopathy introduces unique stressors that can exacerbate headaches and impact overall well-being. Developing a personalized stress-reduction routine is crucial, not only for alleviating headache symptoms but also for improving survivors' and caregivers' quality of life. While stress cannot be entirely avoided, managing it effectively can prevent it from intensifying post-traumatic headaches and other complications.

Identifying Stressors and Tailoring Strategies

Creating a personalized stress-reduction routine starts with recognizing stressors unique to each individual. These may include loud noises, bright lights, mental fatigue, or emotional challenges. Once these triggers are identified, survivors can implement strategies to address them directly. Techniques like progressive muscle relaxation (PMR) and deep breathing exercises can be powerful tools for managing stress. PMR, which involves tensing and releasing specific muscle groups, reduces muscle tension and promotes relaxation. Consistently practicing these exercises can lead to significant improvements in headache management and mental health.[147]

Integrating Mindfulness and Meditation

Mindfulness meditation is another core component of an effective routine. Meditation has been extensively researched for its ability to reduce stress and enhance neuroplasticity, which is vital for brain injury recovery.[148] Setting aside just a few minutes daily for mindfulness meditation can help create a buffer against stress, fostering greater emotional control and focus. Moreover, meditation encourages a shift in perspective, enabling survivors to approach challenges with a calmer mindset, which is crucial for mitigating headaches. Guided meditation programs, accessible through apps or community resources, can be a helpful starting point for beginners.

Engaging in Relaxing Hobbies

Incorporating hobbies into daily life provides a therapeutic outlet for reducing stress. Activities such as painting, journaling, gardening, or crafting not only serve as mental respites but also offer a sense of accomplishment and creativity. These hobbies can be particularly beneficial for survivors of brain injury, as they divert attention from pain and stress, promoting relaxation and a sense of fulfillment. For those unsure of where to begin, experimenting with different activities can help uncover a hobby that brings joy and calm.

Physical Activity as Stress Management

Gentle physical activity, such as walking, yoga, or stretching, is a valuable stress-management strategy that also alleviates headaches. Regular exercise releases endorphins, the body's natural stress relievers, while improving mood and sleep quality. Survivors should consult healthcare professionals to develop safe exercise plans tailored to their abilities. For more detailed guidance on incorporating physical activity, refer to **Chapter 8: The Importance of Physical Activity**, which discusses safe exercises and balancing activity levels to avoid overexertion.

Fostering Emotional Resilience

Practicing gratitude is also an impactful way to shift focus away from stressors. A simple exercise like maintaining a gratitude journal or reflecting on positive moments each day can reduce anxiety and foster emotional resilience. Survivors who incorporate this habit often report improved emotional well-being, which indirectly helps in reducing headache frequency.

Professional Support and Low-Cost Resources

For many survivors, professional support is a key element of stress management. Therapists and counselors specializing in brain injury recovery can provide personalized strategies to address unique challenges. Cognitive-behavioral therapy (CBT), for example, is highly effective for restructuring negative thought patterns and building healthier coping mechanisms.[149] Survivors experiencing financial constraints can access low-cost mental health services through community health centers, university counseling programs, or online platforms offering sliding-scale fees. Caregivers can also play a crucial role in connecting survivors with these resources and providing emotional support throughout the process.

Building a Calming Environment
Creating a relaxing environment is another critical step in stress reduction. Adjusting lighting, reducing noise, and incorporating calming elements like soothing scents or soft music can foster a sense of peace. Survivors and caregivers can work together to design spaces that minimize external stressors and enhance relaxation.

Holistic Approaches to Stress Management
An effective stress-reduction routine integrates these elements into a holistic approach. Survivors may need to experiment with various strategies to find what works best for them. Consistency and adaptability are key; routines should evolve as recovery progresses and needs change.

In summary, developing a stress-reduction routine is a dynamic process that empowers survivors and caregivers to manage stress effectively, reduce headache frequency, and improve overall well-being. By integrating mindfulness, physical activity, relaxing hobbies, emotional resilience practices, and professional support, survivors can regain control over their health and pave the way for long-term recovery.

Chapter 9:
The Importance of Physical Activity

Physical activity plays a vital role in managing headaches and improving overall well-being for those recovering from traumatic brain injuries (TBI), mild traumatic brain injuries (mTBI), concussions, and CTE. Incorporating safe exercises into daily routines can significantly reduce headache frequency and intensity by improving blood flow and stimulating the release of endorphins, natural painkillers.[150]

Regular physical activity also contributes to mood stabilization and stress reduction, both of which are key in preventing headache flare-ups.[151](from Modern Migraine, However, finding the right balance is essential as overexertion can inadvertently trigger headaches rather than alleviate them. A gradual and individualized approach, guided by healthcare professionals, helps ensure that exercise remains a beneficial component of recovery without increasing symptoms. [152]

Safe Exercises for Brain Injury Survivors

Physical activity plays a crucial role in the recovery process for individuals who have experienced traumatic brain injury (TBI), mild traumatic brain injury (mTBI), or a concussion. Engaging in safe and structured exercises can help reduce headache frequency, elevate mood, and support overall brain health. However, it's vital to approach exercise with caution and adapt activity levels to meet individual needs, especially during early recovery. Tailoring movement to one's tolerance can prevent symptom flare-ups and support a gradual, sustainable path to healing.

Balancing Rest and Activity

Recovery begins with a delicate balance between rest and activity. According to one set of clinical recommendations,[153] while an initial rest period of 24–48 hours post-injury is beneficial, prolonged rest beyond this period may hinder recovery. Gradual resumption of activity tailored to the individual's tolerance is key, helping to prevent deconditioning and promoting better physical and mental health outcomes. It's particularly important to avoid activities with a high risk of further injury, emphasizing safe, supervised exercises as part of a recovery plan.

Starting with Gentle and Mind-Body Exercises

For many survivors, the fear of exacerbating symptoms through physical activity is real. This fear can be mitigated by starting with low-impact, gentle exercises. Yoga, tai chi, and other mind-body activities have shown promise in supporting recovery. These exercises promote balance, coordination, and mental focus, all while incorporating controlled movements and mindful breathing. Not only do they enhance body awareness, but they also help survivors manage stress, which is often a contributing factor to headaches. These activities are highly adaptable, making them an excellent starting point for survivors at any stage of recovery.

Walking and Aerobic Exercise

Walking is another safe and effective option, suitable for most TBI and concussion survivors. Starting with short, manageable walks in a calm environment can minimize sensory overload while promoting cardiovascular fitness, mood enhancement, and cognitive function. As endurance builds, survivors can increase duration and intensity gradually. For those ready to take on more aerobic activities, controlled aerobic exercises like stationary cycling or elliptical training may be introduced. Studies have shown[150]150 that supervised, low- to moderate-intensity aerobic exercise can reduce persistent symptoms and improve overall recovery.

Incorporating Vestibular and Balance Training
For survivors experiencing vestibular or balance issues, a common consequence of concussions, exercises targeting these impairments can be invaluable. Research[154] highlights the role of vestibular and ocular motor rehabilitation, such as gaze stabilization exercises and balance training, in alleviating symptoms. These exercises can help individuals regain stability and reduce dizziness, enabling safer and more effective engagement in physical activity.

Aquatic Therapy for Low-Impact Recovery
Aquatic therapy offers unique benefits for those with physical limitations or severe symptoms. The buoyancy of water reduces the strain on joints, allowing survivors to perform movements they might find challenging on land. Activities such as swimming or water walking can improve muscle strength, flexibility, and endurance, all while minimizing the risk of injury. For many survivors, aquatic therapy provides a supportive, therapeutic environment for reintroducing physical activity.

Strength Training and Core Stability
Strength training, introduced with care, can be highly beneficial. Light weights and a focus on proper form help prevent injury while building essential muscle groups. Core stability exercises, such as bridging or seated leg lifts, are particularly valuable for improving balance and coordination. As with other forms of exercise, survivors should start gradually and work under the guidance of a healthcare professional.

Creating a Sustainable Exercise Routine
The goal is to create a sustainable exercise routine that balances activity with rest and aligns with the survivor's unique needs and capabilities. A flexible approach is essential, as recovery is not linear and symptoms can vary daily. Tools like headache diaries can be helpful for tracking the effects of exercise on headache patterns, enabling adjustments to maximize benefits.

The Role of Supervised Programs
Supervised exercise programs are particularly beneficial for individuals with persistent symptoms. Structured activities overseen by healthcare professionals,[153] not only provide physical benefits but also offer psychological reassurance. These programs can help survivors build confidence in their abilities, fostering a positive outlook on recovery.

Tailoring Exercise for Optimal Results
Incorporating evidence-based recommendations,[154] survivors can benefit from tailored approaches to exercise that address specific symptoms, including vestibular dysfunction and headache triggers. Professional guidance ensures that exercises are not only safe but also targeted toward the survivor's unique recovery needs.

Looking Ahead in Chapter 8
The importance of physical activity extends beyond symptom management. In the following sections, we'll explore how exercise directly impacts headache frequency and discuss strategies for balancing activity levels to avoid overexertion. By understanding the physiological and psychological benefits of exercise, survivors can build a comprehensive recovery plan that empowers them to reclaim their quality of life.

How Physical Activity Reduces Headache Frequency

Recovering from a traumatic brain injury (TBI), mild traumatic brain injury (mTBI), concussion, or chronic traumatic encephalopathy (CTE) often involves addressing an unwelcome companion—post-traumatic headaches. For many survivors, these headaches become frequent and debilitating, hindering daily activities and slowing recovery. Interestingly, incorporating safe physical activity into one's routine can serve as a powerful tool to reduce the frequency and severity of these headaches. While it might seem counterintuitive to move while experiencing pain, a growing body of research supports the therapeutic benefits of exercise in headache management.

Physical activity influences the brain in several positive ways, beginning with the enhancement of blood circulation. When you engage in exercise, your heart pumps more efficiently, improving blood flow throughout your body, including the brain. This increased circulation can help reduce headache frequency by ensuring that your brain tissues receive adequate oxygen and nutrients. Additionally, regular physical activity helps control inflammation, a significant factor that can exacerbate headaches after brain injuries. Exercise has been shown to stimulate anti-inflammatory pathways, including the HSP70/NF-κB/IL-6 axis, which can mitigate the chronic inflammation often associated with post-traumatic headaches.[155]

Beyond physical benefits, exercise also plays a significant role in altering our brain chemistry. Activities such as walking, swimming, or yoga stimulate the release of endorphins—our body's natural painkillers. These endorphins interact with the receptors in your brain to reduce the perception of pain. While this is beneficial for everyone, these natural analgesics can be particularly helpful for survivors of TBI, mTBI, or concussion who are experiencing headache pain, providing a non-pharmacological means of relief.[156]

Exercise also supports neural repair and synaptic function, contributing to brain health and recovery. The stimulation of pathways like synapsin I, as highlighted in preclinical studies, suggests that physical activity fosters neuroprotection and resilience following brain injuries. Although these findings stem from animal models, they provide an essential foundation for understanding how exercise might benefit individuals recovering from TBI, mTBI, or concussion.[155]

Additionally, physical activity helps regulate stress and anxiety levels, two common triggers of headaches. When you're active, your brain releases neurotransmitters such as serotonin and dopamine, often called the "feel-good" chemicals. These chemicals not only lift moods but also help dampen stress responses. Given that stress is a significant trigger for headaches, finding effective ways to manage it is crucial for anyone recovering from a brain injury, including those with TBI, mTBI, concussion, or CTE.[157]

Establishing a routine that includes safe and suitable exercises is vital. It's important for brain injury survivors, including those with TBI, mTBI, or concussion, to engage in low-impact exercises that won't overstrain the brain or body. Activities like walking, gentle cycling, or swimming can be contracted into manageable segments throughout the day. This strategy helps avoid overexertion, which can exacerbate symptoms instead of relieving them. Consulting with healthcare professionals to tailor an exercise plan can further ensure safety and effectiveness.

Another benefit of regular exercise is the improvement of sleep patterns, which is crucial for headache management. Physical activity can help regulate your sleep-wake cycles, contributing to better sleep quality, factors directly linked to reduced headache frequency and severity. Inadequate sleep often worsens headaches, so addressing these sleep disturbances through exercise becomes a key part of a holistic management plan.[158]

While the benefits of exercise are evident, it's vital to listen to your body and adjust your activities accordingly. Some days may warrant rest or gentle stretching, especially during a headache flare-up. Balance is key in physical activity to ensure it remains a helpful and not harmful element in headache management.

Despite the challenges of living with a brain injury, it's empowering to know that something as accessible as physical activity can offer relief. Through consistent movement and mindfulness of bodily cues, TBI, mTBI, concussion, and CTE survivors can gain one more tool in their arsenal against headaches, leading to an improved quality of life.

Balancing Activity Levels to Avoid Overexertion

Physical activity stands as a cornerstone for recovery and rehabilitation following brain injuries. Yet, for survivors and their caregivers, one of the fundamental challenges lies in managing the level of physical exertion to ensure it aids rather than hinders progress. The body's response to exercise post-injury can be unpredictable. Overexertion may exacerbate symptoms, including headaches, while appropriate activities can significantly aid recovery. Understanding how to balance activity levels is crucial for improving quality of life after a brain injury.

It's essential to start by recognizing the body's signals. Post-injury, individuals might not have the same stamina or threshold for physical stress as they did before. Symptoms such as increased headache, dizziness, or fatigue during or after physical activity can signal overexertion.[159] By acknowledging these signals, survivors and their caretakers can tailor activity levels to avoid adverse effects, allowing for a more sustainable integration of physical activity into recovery routines.

Adopting a gradual approach to physical activity is recommended. This involves starting with low-intensity exercises and slowly increasing duration and intensity as tolerated. Activities such as walking, stationary biking, or swimming are often recommended due to their low-impact nature.[160] Controlled aerobic exercise has been shown to restore cerebral blood flow, reduce symptoms, and support neurometabolic recovery—particularly in individuals with concussions, but emerging evidence suggests benefits for other forms of brain injury as well, including TBI and mTBI. Moreover, the mental health benefits of exercise, including reduced anxiety and improved mood, are particularly valuable for those managing post-concussion symptoms. This underscores the importance of individualized exercise prescriptions guided by symptom monitoring and recovery progress.

Preconditioning exercises, as supported by research, can build resilience against overexertion and support long-term recovery.[155] Careful monitoring of response to each increment in activity level is key. Individuals should aim for consistency and gradual progress rather than rapid increases that could lead to setbacks.

Incorporating structured exercise plans that combine aerobic activities, strength training, and neuro-rehabilitation exercises can significantly enhance recovery from brain injuries. Such comprehensive programs address multiple facets of physical health, promoting overall well-being.

For instance, the UPMC Sports Medicine Concussion Program outlines a five-stage rehabilitation protocol that progressively increases physical exertion levels. This protocol includes aerobic exercises, sport-specific activities, and non-contact training drills, ensuring a balanced approach to recovery.[161]

Similarly, a study published in the Journal of Neuroinflammation highlights how exercise can modulate inflammatory responses and protect against neurological deficits following TBI. The findings suggest that exercise preconditioning can reduce inflammation and improve outcomes after TBI by stimulating specific anti-inflammatory pathways. [155]

These structured programs are tailored to individual recovery needs, emphasizing the importance of personalized exercise prescriptions. By integrating various exercise modalities, they offer a comprehensive strategy to support physical and neurological rehabilitation.

Integrating rest periods is another critical element. Contrary to some traditional beliefs focusing solely on rest, a combination of rest and controlled activity can yield better outcomes.[162] The balance between activity and rest ensures the body has the necessary time to recover, helping prevent the worsening of symptoms such as headaches. Listening to the body's need for rest amidst a structured routine is vital for sustainable progress.

Chapter 10:
Medical Treatments and Interventions

In addressing the complex landscape of post-traumatic headaches, medical treatments and interventions provide essential avenues for relief and recovery. A multifaceted approach, grounded in collaboration with healthcare professionals, can significantly enhance patient outcomes. Medications such as non-steroidal anti-inflammatory drugs (NSAIDs) and triptans are frequently prescribed to mitigate headache symptoms, while newer options target specific pathways involved in headache genesis.[163] Physical therapy often plays a role in recovery by promoting muscle relaxation and improving posture, which can alleviate tension-type headaches exacerbated by brain injury.[164] Beyond conventional medicine, alternative therapies like acupuncture and biofeedback have shown promise in reducing headache frequency and intensity, though their efficacy can vary from person to person.[165] Therefore, tailoring treatment plans to individual needs, and maintaining open communication with your healthcare team, is paramount in navigating the road to recovery.

Medications Commonly Used for Post-Traumatic Headaches

Managing post-traumatic headaches is a complex challenge for many individuals recovering from traumatic brain injury (TBI), mild TBI (mTBI), concussion, or chronic traumatic encephalopathy (CTE). While lifestyle changes and non-medical interventions play a significant role, medications often provide essential relief. Understanding the options available and knowing how they work can empower patients and caregivers to make informed decisions in collaboration with healthcare providers.

Pharmacological treatments for post-traumatic headaches are often divided into two categories: abortive and preventive medications. Abortive treatments are used to alleviate the headache as it occurs, while preventive medications aim to reduce the frequency and severity of headaches over time. Recognizing which category a medication falls into is crucial for managing symptoms effectively.

Abortive Medications

Abortive medications are taken at the onset of a headache to stop it from advancing. Nonsteroidal anti-inflammatory drugs (NSAIDs) like ibuprofen and naproxen are commonly used for their efficacy in reducing inflammation and pain. While these over-the-counter options are accessible and effective, overuse can lead to rebound headaches, where excessive medication use paradoxically increases headache frequency. Research highlights that while NSAIDs may have protective effects against migraine progression when used appropriately, their overuse can exacerbate the risk of chronic headache development.[166]

For more severe or chronic cases, prescription medications such as triptans might be recommended. Triptans, including sumatriptan and rizatriptan, work by promoting serotonin levels, which helps to constrict blood vessels and reduce inflammation in the brain. While effective, triptans are generally reserved for cases that do not respond to NSAIDs or in individuals where migraines are a dominant component of their post-traumatic headache profile.[167]

Another class of abortive medication is the ergotamines, like ergotamine tartrate. These drugs also narrow blood vessels around the brain, but they're typically used less frequently due to their potential side effects and contraindications. The effectiveness of the ergotamines can vary, and they are not suitable for everyone, particularly due to their potential interaction with other medications.[168]

Preventive Medications
Preventive medications are taken regularly, often daily, to reduce headache frequency and severity. Beta-blockers, such as propranolol and metoprolol, are one of the most well-known classes of preventives for migraine headaches, including post-traumatic types. These medications reduce the workload of the heart and influence blood vessel dilation, helping to manage migraines by stabilizing vascular activity. Studies have demonstrated their efficacy in reducing the frequency and severity of migraines, making them a cornerstone of preventive treatment.[169]

Antidepressants, particularly tricyclics like amitriptyline, are another option. They work by altering neurotransmitter levels in the brain, reducing headache symptoms for some patients. Antidepressants can also address co-occurring depression or anxiety, offering dual benefits in symptom management.[170] However, these medications require careful monitoring to manage potential side effects, such as drowsiness or weight gain.

Anticonvulsants like topiramate and valproate have also demonstrated efficacy in reducing headache frequency among those with post-traumatic headaches. These medications stabilize neural pathways, preventing the onset of headache episodes. While beneficial, anticonvulsants can have side effects, including cognitive impacts and nausea, necessitating close consultation with healthcare providers for tailored treatment plans.[170]

Emerging Medications and Their Role
Botulinum toxin (Botox) injections have been explored as a treatment for chronic migraines and, by extension, post-traumatic headache sufferers. The toxin works by blocking neurotransmitter release responsible for inflammation and pain perception. A study on military veterans demonstrated the potential efficacy of botulinum toxin type A in reducing the frequency and severity of post-traumatic headaches, especially in chronic cases. This randomized, placebo-controlled study supports the use of Botox as an alternative for individuals who do not respond to conventional treatments.[171]

CGRP (Calcitonin Gene-Related Peptide) monoclonal antibodies represent another promising treatment option on the horizon. Drugs like erenumab and fremanezumab target the proteins involved in migraine pathology, potentially providing relief for those with a migraine-heavy profile in their post-traumatic headaches. Recent research highlights the successful translation of CGRP-targeting therapies from bench to clinic, showing significant reductions in headache frequency for many patients.[172] Though relatively new, these treatments offer hope for more targeted headache management strategies in the future.

Considerations and Consultations

When it comes to choosing a medication, a personalized approach is vital. What works for one person may not work for another due to the variability in symptoms, individual health conditions, and underlying headache triggers. The concept of personalized medicine in headache management underscores tailoring treatment strategies to biochemical profiles, comorbidities, and patient history.[173] Collaboration with a healthcare provider ensures a treatment plan that is both safe and effective.

Side effects remain a critical aspect of any medication discussion. Adverse effects must always be balanced against the anticipated benefits. Research into emerging therapies highlights the need for ongoing monitoring and adjustments to treatment plans, emphasizing patient-provider communication as a cornerstone of successful management.[174]

In the end, while medications are a crucial tool in managing post-traumatic headaches, they are most effective when combined with lifestyle adjustments such as sleep optimization, stress reduction, nutrition, and physical activity. As research progresses, innovative medications like CGRP inhibitors and novel uses for botulinum toxin offer renewed hope for more effective headache management strategies.

Physical Therapy and Alternative Therapies

For individuals recovering from brain injuries - including traumatic brain injury (TBI), mild TBI (mTBI), concussion, or chronic traumatic encephalopathy (CTE) - managing post-traumatic headaches often requires a multifaceted approach. While medications and lifestyle changes are important, therapies such as physical therapy, acupuncture, chiropractic care, biofeedback, and mind-body practices offer complementary pathways to recovery. These treatments support neurological healing and symptom relief through physical movement, nervous system regulation, and stress reduction.

Research supports the integration of these approaches into comprehensive care plans. Physical therapy can improve posture and relieve neck-related tension; manual therapy and acupuncture reduce muscle strain and promote circulation; and yoga, biofeedback, and meditation target stress and pain perception at the neurological level. This section explores the science and practical applications of these strategies, helping survivors, caregivers, and healthcare professionals consider effective non-pharmacological tools to reduce headache burden and enhance daily functioning.

Physical Therapy's Role in Recovery

Physical therapy (PT) is an essential part of recovery for many brain injury survivors. The primary goal of PT is to restore movement, improve physical function, and reduce pain. For headache sufferers, PT can involve specific exercises that target the neck and shoulders, regions often contributing to headache symptoms. By improving mobility and flexibility in these areas, physical therapy can help alleviate tension and stress that might lead to headaches.

The role of the physical therapist extends beyond prescribing exercises. They provide education on body mechanics, posture, and ergonomic principles. Research highlights that maintaining proper posture can significantly decrease headache frequency and intensity. Additionally, understanding and practicing safe movement techniques help prevent re-injury and manage existing symptoms effectively (Fernández-de-las-Peñas et al. (2007) [175].

Manual Therapy for Headache Relief

One common modality employed in PT is manual therapy. This hands-on technique involves gentle manipulation of soft tissues and joints. Research suggests manual therapy can significantly reduce headache frequency and intensity by relieving muscle tension and improving circulation)[176]. Moreover, it fosters a sense of relaxation and promotes the well-being of patients, enhancing their recovery journey.

Alternative Therapies for Holistic Support

Alternative therapies, although less conventional, have shown promise in managing post-traumatic headaches. Acupuncture, for instance, has gained credibility as a complementary treatment for headache relief. By stimulating specific points in the body, acupuncture can help restore balance in the nervous system and reduce headache symptoms

(Vickers et al., 2012)[177]. Many patients report short-term relief and a decrease in headache severity after regular sessions.

Chiropractic care, another alternative therapy, focuses on diagnosing and treating mechanical disorders of the musculoskeletal system, particularly the spine. Evidence-based guidelines suggest that chiropractic spinal manipulation may offer relief to those suffering from headaches, particularly if they stem from neck issues (Bryans et al., 2011)[178]. However, it's crucial for anyone considering chiropractic treatment to consult with a healthcare provider to ensure it's appropriate for their specific condition.

Biofeedback is another alternative approach gaining traction in headache management. This technique involves learning to control physiological processes such as muscle tension and heart rate through real-time data feedback. Biofeedback can empower patients to manage their stress response and potentially decrease headache occurrence. Studies show that with consistent practice, biofeedback may effectively reduce headache frequency and severity.[179]

Yoga and Meditation for Mind-Body Connection

Yoga and meditation shouldn't be overlooked as valuable tools for headache management. These practices train the body and mind to engage in deep relaxation and mindfulness. Yoga, in particular, strengthens muscles, improves posture, and teaches breathing techniques, all of which are beneficial in managing headaches. Meditation aids in reducing stress and anxiety levels, directly impacting headache frequency. Regular practice of these disciplines can lead to substantial improvements in pain perception and overall quality of life.[180]

Integrated Approaches for Comprehensive Care

It's essential to recognize that integrating these therapies requires a holistic and coordinated approach. Collaborating with healthcare professionals ensures that treatments are tailored to meet the individual's needs, considering all aspects of their physical and mental health. This collaborative effort involves open communication among different practitioners, including doctors, physical therapists, acupuncturists, and chiropractors, ensuring cohesive and effective treatment plans.

Finally, while these alternative therapies can provide significant benefits, they may not be a standalone solution for everyone. It's vital for survivors and caregivers to balance these treatments with other medical interventions, medication when necessary, and lifestyle adjustments mentioned in previous chapters. Being proactive in exploring various therapies and remaining committed to the treatment plan can enhance recovery and manage headaches more effectively.

The journey to managing headaches post-brain injury is highly personal, and finding the right combination of therapies requires patience and persistence. Survivors and their caregivers should approach these treatments with an open mind, considering what aligns best with their values and lifestyle. While the road may seem arduous, embracing a comprehensive approach that includes physical therapy and alternative treatments can make a significant difference in achieving long-term relief and improving overall well-being.

Collaborating with Healthcare Professionals for Customized Treatment

Finding effective relief for post-traumatic headaches isn't a one-size-fits-all endeavor. Survivors of traumatic brain injuries—including TBI, mTBI, concussion, and CTE—require a tailored approach that meticulously considers their unique medical histories, symptoms, and circumstances. Collaborating with healthcare professionals is crucial to building a personalized treatment plan that addresses the specific needs of each individual. This partnership isn't merely about following medical advice; it's about active engagement in the treatment process, fostering an environment where your voice is heard and respected.

One of the first steps in working with healthcare professionals is identifying the right team of experts. This team can include neurologists, physiatrists, physical therapists, psychologists, and even dietitians, each bringing their own expertise to create a comprehensive treatment strategy. A multidisciplinary approach has been shown to be particularly effective in treating complex headache disorders, as it fosters collaboration among various specialists to address different facets of headache management.[181]

Communication plays a pivotal role in this process. Being open about your symptoms, triggers, and how they impact your daily life can provide invaluable information for healthcare practitioners. Conveying how you feel in a clear and comprehensive manner allows professionals to formulate interventions that are closely aligned with your experiences. This input is critical, as it provides the foundation upon which the treatment plan is built. It's also important to express any concerns or questions you might have about recommended therapies or medications, helping to adjust the plan as needed.

In this collaborative dynamic, it's beneficial to be well-informed about the latest research, treatment options, and resources for post-traumatic headaches. Staying informed allows survivors and caregivers to engage in meaningful discussions with their healthcare team and advocate for the best possible care. Here's a summary of recent findings and valuable resources:

Latest Research

- **Frequency and Predictors of Headache:** A study published in *The Journal of Headache and Pain* highlights that headaches are a prevalent and debilitating symptom following traumatic brain injury (TBI). Factors such as younger age, more severe TBI, fatigue, neck pain, and vision problems were found to predict more severe headaches over time.

- **Emerging Treatment Options:** A review in *Current Pain and Headache Reports* evaluated evidence-based treatments for post-traumatic headaches (PTH). Acute treatments include medications like metoclopramide with diphenhydramine, while persistent cases have responded to newer therapies such as erenumab. Non-drug treatments like cognitive-behavioral therapy and transcranial magnetic stimulation also hold promise.

Updated Treatment Guidelines

- **American Headache Society:** Clinical guidelines emphasize the use of calcitonin gene-related peptide (CGRP)-targeting therapies as a first-line option for prevention of post-traumatic headaches.

- **UpToDate:** This comprehensive resource offers guidelines on the epidemiology, clinical features, treatment, and prognosis of post-traumatic headaches, providing actionable insights for both patients and providers.

Patient Advocacy and Support Websites

- **National Headache Foundation:** Offers a wealth of resources for patients, including tips on accessing care, reducing stigma, and advocating for support.

- **American Migraine Foundation:** Provides detailed information on post-traumatic headaches, including types, symptoms, and treatment options, tailored to empower patients and caregivers.

By discussing these findings and resources with your healthcare professionals, you can explore how they might integrate into your treatment plan. Being proactive and informed not only enhances communication but also fosters collaboration, ensuring that the strategies employed are both effective and tailored to your needs.

Another advantage of collaboration is the potential to explore a variety of treatment modalities. Medications are a primary intervention, yet they're often just one part of a larger strategy. As reviewed, alternative therapies, such as acupuncture, biofeedback, and cognitive-behavioral therapy, have been shown to complement traditional treatments and enhance outcomes.[182] While some of these methods are still being researched for their efficacy in headache treatment, discussing their potential use with your healthcare provider can lead to innovative and custom-tailored regimens .

It's also vital to ensure that the treatment plan developed with healthcare professionals is adaptable. As your circumstances change, or new treatments become available, your plan should be flexible enough to accommodate these developments. Regular follow-up appointments offer opportunities to review the plan's effectiveness and make adjustments as needed. This iterative process can help in managing symptoms more effectively and adjusting the approach as your condition evolves.

Collaboration extends beyond simply attending appointments. It involves an active partnership, where both you and your healthcare provider continually engage in discussions about progress and setbacks. This ongoing dialogue ensures that treatment remains relevant and effective in meeting your needs. Keeping a headache diary can also facilitate these conversations by providing concrete data on headache frequency, triggers, and lifestyle impacts, offering insight into how various treatments are working.[181]

Finally, involving family members or caregivers in discussions with healthcare professionals can further enrich the collaborative process. They can provide additional insights into your struggles and successes, and offer support in implementing treatment plans tailored for you. Plus, having a dependable support system can mitigate stress, which is known to exacerbate headache symptoms.[183]

Collaborating with healthcare professionals paves the way for a customized treatment plan that acknowledges the complexities of post-traumatic headaches. By embracing a multi-disciplinary approach coupled with active personal engagement, the journey toward finding relief becomes a shared commitment. Empowered with knowledge and supported by professionals, patients can navigate the path to improved quality of life and sustained well-being.

Chapter 11:
Lifestyle Adjustments for Headache Prevention

Continuing our exploration into improving the quality of life for individuals with brain injuries—including TBI, mTBI, concussion, and CTE—this chapter focuses on how lifestyle adjustments can play a pivotal role in preventing headaches. Implementing consistent daily routines tailored to individual needs can stabilize the body's circadian rhythms, often disrupted post-injury, which in turn supports headache prevention. Identifying and avoiding specific triggers, such as certain foods or environmental factors, is crucial.[184] Fostering a supportive environment at home, school, or work further reinforces recovery by acknowledging the challenges of life after brain injury and encouraging consistency.[185] Fostering a supportive environment at home, school, or work further reinforces recovery by acknowledging the challenges of life after brain injury and encouraging consistency.[186]

Creating Daily Routines That Support Headache Prevention

For individuals recovering from brain injuries—including TBI, mTBI, concussion, or CTE—designing a daily routine that reduces the likelihood of headache triggers is essential. Establishing predictable schedules for waking, sleeping, eating, and rest not only reinforces physical recovery but also improves emotional regulation and energy levels. A structured routine provides a sense of control-something often lost after a brain injury - and helps survivors better manage the unpredictability of post-traumatic headaches.

The first step in crafting a headache-preventive routine is understanding individual triggers. Keeping a headache diary enables survivors and their caregivers to identify patterns that may contribute to headache onsets, such as specific activities, foods, or stressors.[187] This information is invaluable in creating a personalized prevention strategy tailored to the individual's unique needs.

Consistency is key in routine establishment. Wake-up and bedtimes should remain constant even on weekends, as irregular sleep schedules are known to exacerbate headaches.[188] Morning routines might include gentle stretching or short periods of meditation to promote relaxation and set a positive tone for the day. These low-intensity activities can help ease tension that might lead to headaches, particularly for those with a history of head trauma.

An integral aspect of these routines is incorporating balanced nutrition. Consistent meal times and a diet rich in whole grains, lean proteins, and plenty of fruits and vegetables provide the necessary nutrients and sustained energy levels throughout the day. Fluctuating blood sugar can trigger headaches; therefore, regular meal schedules are critical.[189] Morning meals can be simple but should never be skipped. A mix of proteins and carbohydrates can be particularly effective in maintaining energy without causing spikes.

Hydration plays a vital role in headache prevention. Dehydration is a common trigger for headaches, and individuals should aim to drink water consistently throughout the day. Small interventions like carrying a reusable water bottle can prompt more frequent sips and make hydrating easier. Recognizing signs of thirst and adapting intake are essential parts of structuring a daily routine around headache prevention.[189]

As the day progresses, it's important to integrate short breaks to alleviate potential stress led by continuous activities or screen time. Scheduling brief but frequent breaks can mitigate tension buildup and prevent headaches associated with prolonged physical or cognitive strain. These breaks provide opportunities to reset before diving back into tasks, reducing stress and promoting mental clarity.

Incorporating physical activity is another vital element. While it's essential to engage in safe, exercise-tailored to each individual's recovery stage, even light movements can enhance overall well-being. Activities like walking, gentle yoga, or tai chi can increase oxygen flow and improve mood, both of which are beneficial in managing headaches.[187] These should be planned for times when energy levels are typically higher, such as mid-morning or early afternoon, depending on personal patterns.

Evening routines should focus on winding down. Dimming lights, reducing electronics usage, and engaging in calming activities can prepare the body for sleep and reduce the likelihood of nighttime headaches. Techniques such as deep-breathing exercises, light reading, or listening to calming music can be effective tools to transition from a busy day to a restful night. Creating a bedtime ritual signals the brain to prepare for sleep, a crucial component of headache prevention.[188]

Lastly, it's paramount to remember flexibility in daily routines. While structure is beneficial, rigid schedules can become overwhelming and contribute to stress. Listening to one's body and making adjustments as necessary can enhance the effectiveness of these routines and prevent them from becoming a source of anxiety.

Recovery from brain injuries is multifaceted, and while daily routines can provide significant support, they must evolve with the individual's progress and lifestyle changes. Caregivers can play a pivotal role by helping to maintain consistency while allowing room for adjustments. Engaging with medical professionals to continually assess and refine routines ensures they align well with the ongoing recovery and health goals.

Creating routines focused on headache prevention is an empowering step toward regaining control over one's life after a brain injury. By weaving together aspects of relaxation, nutrition, physical activity, and flexibility, individuals can construct a daily scaffold that not only supports headache prevention but also enhances overall quality of life.

Identifying and Avoiding Headache Triggers

Understanding and avoiding headache triggers is a key strategy in minimizing the frequency and intensity of headaches for those coping with traumatic brain injury (TBI), concussions, or chronic traumatic encephalopathy (CTE). It's a process that calls for vigilance, experimentation, and patience, but the payoff can be a significant improvement in quality of life. What makes this an essential topic is the individuality of headache triggers; what sets off a headache for one person may not affect another. By identifying personal triggers, individuals can make informed decisions to prevent future headaches. This section outlines some common triggers and offers practical advice on how to avoid them.

Environmental factors rank high among headache triggers, often referred to as sensory overload in TBI survivors. Keeping a detailed headache diary to track potential environmental exposures before a headache begins can help identify specific triggers, such as bright lights or loud noises.[190] Over time, this process can reveal patterns and inform strategies to avoid these stimuli.

Dietary triggers such as aged cheese, alcohol, and MSG are common culprits. While some individuals may find caffeine helpful in moderation, others experience withdrawal headaches or sensitivity from excessive intake. Testing dietary changes incrementally allows individuals to isolate problematic foods and manage headache frequency effectively.[191] Regular meals to stabilize blood sugar levels also play a vital role.

Stress management is essential, as chronic stress exacerbates headaches through physiological mechanisms like muscle tension and hormonal shifts. Mindfulness practices, structured relaxation periods, or even gentle breathing exercises can help mitigate stress-induced headaches.[192] Incorporating these tools into daily routines provides a proactive means of reducing headache frequency.

Sleep disturbances frequently contribute to headache onset. Establishing consistent sleep routines and creating a calming sleep environment are particularly beneficial for TBI survivors.

Relaxation aids such as white noise machines or guided meditation can facilitate restful sleep, minimizing this significant trigger.[193]

Another angle to consider involves hormonal fluctuations, especially relevant to women. Hormonal changes such as those experienced during menstrual cycles, pregnancy, or menopause can significantly impact headache frequency and severity. Keeping track of such patterns in a headache diary can provide insights that are useful when discussing management strategies with healthcare providers.

Physical exertion might also act as a trigger, particularly high-intensity or high-impact activities. TBI and concussion survivors need to find a balance between maintaining physical activity for overall health and avoiding activities that could induce headaches. It's worth experimenting with different types and intensities of exercise to identify what feels manageable and minimize headache occurrence. Activities like walking, tai chi, or gentle yoga can be useful as they typically don't exert as much strain.

Lastly, regular consultations with healthcare providers can offer personalized guidance on identifying and navigating potential headache triggers. They might suggest modifications to daily routines or recommend medical interventions where lifestyle adjustments alone aren't fully effective. Collaborating with medical professionals ensures a well-rounded approach to headache prevention tailored to the specific needs of TBI, concussion, and CTE survivors.

Armed with the insights gained from identifying headache triggers, individuals can make proactive changes that will help reduce headache frequency and severity. It's about creating an environment—both physical and emotional—that supports recovery and minimizes stressors. With time, patience, and persistence, many find that their journey through this process leads not only to fewer headaches but also to an improved sense of overall well-being.

Building a Supportive Environment for Recovery

Creating a supportive environment is crucial for individuals recovering from brain injuries and managing post-traumatic headaches. Often overlooked, the physical and emotional spaces we inhabit can significantly influence our healing process and overall well-being. An environment that's tailored to the needs of someone recovering from TBI can make a tangible difference in their quality of life, aiding in faster and more effective headache relief.

A supportive recovery environment begins with ensuring physical safety and comfort at home. The living space should be safe and accessible, minimizing any potential hazards that may exacerbate symptoms or lead to accidents. For instance, ensuring that walkways are clear and lighting is adequate can prevent trips and falls, which might otherwise provoke or worsen headaches. For those with heightened sensitivity to light, incorporating soft, adjustable lighting throughout the home can be particularly beneficial.[194]

Equally important is fostering an emotionally supportive atmosphere. Caregivers who understand the nuances of TBI and headache management can provide meaningful support. Empathy and communication reduce stress levels, a crucial factor in headache prevention.[195] Open discussions about symptoms and challenges allow families to adapt routines and minimize triggers proactively.

Communication is another cornerstone of a supportive recovery environment. Establishing open channels of communication within the household helps survivors express their needs and any discomfort they experience. This expression can lead to tailored adjustments in daily activities, thus minimizing headache triggers. Integrating regular family meetings or check-ins can be effective ways to ensure everyone is on the same page and to anticipate the survivor's needs before they become pressing issues.

In addition to social support, the home environment should foster rest and relaxation. A peaceful and quiet space designated for recovery can make a significant difference. This area should be free of unnecessary noise and comfortable enough to encourage rest. It might be beneficial to designate a quiet room with calming colors and soothing sounds, promoting relaxation and aiding in stress reduction.

Sensory sensitivities, such as heightened reactivity to noise or smells, also need consideration. Soundproofing solutions and scent-free environments can significantly benefit survivors.[194] These adjustments reduce stressors that might otherwise exacerbate headaches.

Technology can also play a role in building a supportive environment. Smart home devices, like lights that adjust automatically based on the time of day or ambient conditions, can reduce effort and cognitive strain. Apps and devices that track daily routines can help remember medication schedules, appointments, and other therapeutic activities without adding cognitive burden, which can otherwise lead to increased headache frequency.

Another key element to consider is the integration of activities that promote both mental and physical well-being. Encouraging hobbies and interests that the survivor enjoys can provide a much-needed mental break. Tailoring these activities to one's abilities and fatigue levels is important to prevent overexertion, which can be a headache trigger. Simple, low-intensity activities like gardening, gentle craft work, or puzzles can offer mental engagement without causing strain.

Support extends into the community, too. Engaging with local support groups and community resources can provide additional layers of care and understanding. These connections not only help survivors feel less isolated but also offer a platform to share experiences and coping strategies with others facing similar challenges. Members of these groups often share practical advice for modifying environments based on personal experiences, which can offer new insights into managing headaches effectively.

It's essential to include educational resources as part of the environment. Educational books, pamphlets, or materials recommended by healthcare providers can be invaluable. They equip both the survivor and their caregivers with the knowledge to navigate challenges better and provide evidence-based approaches to managing symptoms when they arise. Regularly revisiting these resources can keep the information fresh and applicable.

Building a supportive environment is a dynamic, continuous process, requiring adjustments as recovery progresses. These changes should be compassionate and considerate of the survivor's current needs, which can fluctuate day by day. By prioritizing safety, sensory management, communication, emotional support, and community connection, the environment itself becomes a reliable ally in the journey toward recovery.

Ultimately, developing an environment that supports recovery involves both physical arrangements and emotional nurturance. Both elements can profoundly impact headache management and overall quality of life, and are just as valuable as any medical or therapeutic intervention. This comprehensive approach ensures that the survivor is surrounded by a network of support, fostering resilience and hope on the path to recovery.

Chapter 12:
Building Your Support System

Creating a strong support system is crucial for navigating the ups and downs of life after a traumatic brain injury, concussion, or CTE. Leaning on family, friends, and caregivers can make a significant difference in managing the challenges that come with post-traumatic headaches. Open and honest communication is key to ensuring those around you understand your needs, whether that means seeking help with daily tasks or simply having someone to listen to when the load feels heavy. Additionally, joining support groups, whether in-person or online, offers a sense of community and shared experiences that can be invaluable. Such groups provide not only emotional support but also practical advice and tips from others who truly get what you're going through.[196] Engaging with people who are walking a similar path can foster a sense of belonging and empower you to take greater control over your health journey. Remember, building this network isn't just about asking for help; it's also about celebrating victories big and small, fostering resilience, and developing strategies to improve overall well-being.

Seeking Support from Family, Friends, and Caregivers

Building a support system is crucial for individuals recovering from traumatic brain injuries (TBI), concussions, and chronic traumatic encephalopathy (CTE). It's a journey populated by different needs, fears, and hopes that can be overwhelming at times. But one of the most pivotal elements in navigating this journey is the encouragement and assistance from family, friends, and caregivers. This network not only provides emotional comfort but also practical help that energy-sapped individuals may need to regain their footing.

Close relationships bear the potential to offer a compassionate buffer against the ripple effects of recurring headaches, mood changes, and physical limitations that often accompany brain injuries. Friends and family can extend their support in numerous ways, starting from small, everyday tasks such as preparing meals, running errands, or accompanying the survivor to medical appointments. These acts alleviate stress and provide the survivor more mental bandwidth to focus on their recovery journey.

Equally important is emotional support, which can dramatically improve mental well-being. Having someone to talk to, share experiences with, or simply be present in times of distress can mitigate feelings of isolation and loneliness that frequently beset those paving their path to recovery. Emotional support also engages the brain's "safety" mechanisms, which can lower stress levels and thus reduce headache frequency and intensity.[197]

Family and friends also play a role in understanding the unique triggers and symptoms that manifest in the wake of a head injury. Observant partners can notice patterns in headache triggers, such as specific foods, activities, or stress triggers, that the survivor might overlook. By being attuned to these signals, families can help in tracking headache patterns and adjusting routines or environments to minimize discomfort, making daily life more manageable.

Communication is essential in these relationships. Survivors benefit significantly when they express their needs openly and clearly. Misunderstandings are less likely, and conversations can shift toward actionable solutions, whether that's rearranging a particularly bustling routine or exploring new therapies. Practical advice for improving communication, such as using clear, open dialogue and overcoming common communication barriers, can help caregivers better understand and support their loved ones during recovery.[198] Effective communication fosters a shared understanding and strengthens the caregiver-survivor bond, paving the way for smoother collaboration and better outcomes.

For caregivers, taking care of someone with a brain injury can be equally challenging. Feelings of compassion fatigue or burnout are common as they juggle the dual roles of caring for others and maintaining their personal lives. Therefore, it's essential for caregivers to build their own support systems, whether through professional counseling or community groups tailored to their experiences. Ensuring that the caregiver's mental health is also addressed can sustain the quality of care provided to TBI survivors. The reciprocal exchange of support leads to a fortified support system where everyone thrives.

Finally, involving family and friends early in the recovery process can have potential long-term benefits. Studies show that social interactions and strong networks are linked to better health outcomes and increased quality of life.[199] Community involvement or participation in social activities can offer a sense of normalcy and belonging, contributing positively to the healing process.

For all parties involved, education about TBI and headaches can demystify many of the challenges faced, fostering empathy and enhancing care. Educational workshops and materials prepared by medical professionals can arm family and friends with practical knowledge to offer better-informed support. This collective understanding allows for more nuanced care, prioritizing the survivor's health and well-being.

To conclude, building a reliable support system is not a one-way street but a cooperative venture among the survivor and family, friends, and caregivers. By pooling emotional strength and practical assistance, TBI survivors can create a nurturing environment that bolsters their healing journey while simultaneously enriching their relationships.

Communicating Your Needs Effectively

Building a robust support system can significantly aid the healing process for individuals recovering from traumatic brain injuries (TBI), concussions, or chronic traumatic encephalopathy (CTE). At the heart of this support system is the vital skill of communicating your needs effectively. Whether you are a survivor, caregiver, or health professional, understanding how to articulate needs clearly can be a game-changer in managing post-traumatic headaches and enhancing overall quality of life.

The challenge of expressing needs effectively often arises from a combination of physical discomfort and emotional hurdles. A brain injury can sometimes affect not just cognitive abilities but also the emotions connected with communication. It's crucial to acknowledge any feelings of frustration, shame, or anxiety that may accompany these interactions. Recognizing these emotions can help in finding the right strategies to express needs constructively.

Start by being specific about your pain and symptoms. A clear description helps convey the severity and specific nature of your headaches. Use simple language to explain your experience. For instance, instead of saying "I don't feel well," try "I'm experiencing a sharp headache that makes it hard to concentrate." Use physical indicators and pain scales, if necessary, to provide a more objective measure of your discomfort.

Non-verbal communication can be just as crucial as verbal communication. Gestures, facial expressions, and even written descriptions can help convey your message more effectively. For many survivors, these can act as alternative forms of expression when verbal communication might be too exhausting or difficult. It's essential for caregivers and family members to be attentive to these non-verbal cues and respond supportively.

An open line of communication with caregivers and healthcare providers can foster mutual understanding and trust. Caregivers, on their part, should actively listen, confirm they understand by asking clarifying questions, and ensure they provide feedback that is empathetic and supportive. Having open-ended conversations where both parties feel heard and respected can contribute significantly to effective communication.

For health professionals, clear documentation in medical records is vital. Maintain detailed records of symptoms and any changes over time, as these will be instrumental in developing and adjusting treatment strategies. Regular consultations with medical professionals should include discussions about all treatment options, as well as lifestyle modifications that may benefit the patient's well-being.

Many survivors find it beneficial to practice communication strategies. This might include role-playing exercises with a therapist or support person to build confidence before having critical discussions about needs and treatment plans. Role-playing provides a safe space to explore various scenarios and responses, ensuring that both the survivor and their support system are well-prepared.

In some cases, technology can serve as an invaluable tool in communicating needs. With the availability of apps and devices specifically designed to aid those with cognitive challenges, expressing needs has become more accessible. These tools offer features such as voice-to-text capabilities, reminder settings, and direct communication functions that can ease some of the burdens of expression.

Building a mutual understanding with those around you can alleviate the stress and anxiety associated with post-traumatic symptoms. It's beneficial to involve family members and caregivers in workshops or informational sessions that highlight the importance of clear communication and understanding the unique challenges faced by brain injury survivors.

Moreover, consider joining support groups. These communities can offer additional insights and strategies for effective communication, fostering a sense of belonging and reducing feelings of isolation. Connecting with others who share similar experiences can provide comfort and encourage open dialogue about managing expectations and needs.

Lastly, be patient with yourself and your progress. Communication is a skill that, like any other, can improve with time and practice. Celebrating small victories and understanding setbacks as part of the journey can lead to a more resilient approach to managing post-traumatic headaches. It's important to recognize the significant role communication plays in building a supportive network and accessing the resources needed for recovery.

By prioritizing effective communication, brain injury survivors, along with their caregivers and healthcare providers, can work towards a more coordinated and compassionate approach to managing health challenges. This effort not only improves health outcomes but also enhances the quality of relationships and, ultimately, the survivor's quality of life.

Finding and Joining Support Groups and Online Communities

Building a robust support system is pivotal for managing headaches after a brain injury. Feeling connected to others who understand your journey can be a source of immense relief and empowerment. Support groups and online communities cater specifically to traumatic brain injury (TBI) survivors, concussion sufferers, and individuals living with chronic traumatic encephalopathy (CTE). Finding the right group can help you learn new coping strategies and provide an empathetic ear when you need it most.

Support groups offer a sense of belonging and community, which is crucial for mental well-being. They can be local, allowing for face-to-face interactions, or virtual, offering flexibility and access from anywhere. Both types have unique benefits. Local groups provide personal interaction and physical comfort, which may resonate more with individuals who prefer seeing facial expressions and reading body cues. Online communities, on the other hand, are convenient and offer anonymity that can encourage more open sharing among members who might be hesitant to talk in person.

The first step in finding a support group is to identify what you hope to achieve by joining. Are you looking for emotional support, practical advice, or information about the latest research and treatment options? Determining your goals can direct you to a group that aligns with your needs. Some groups focus on sharing experiences and emotional support, while others may have regular guest speakers or discuss scientific developments and treatment strategies.

Connecting with a group that addresses your specific condition is essential. Many organizations, such as the Brain Injury Association of America or the Concussion Legacy Foundation, offer directories of TBI- and concussion-specific support groups. These organizations understand the complexities associated with brain injuries and can facilitate connections with experienced peers.

Online communities have burgeoned, especially in an era where digital connectivity plays a significant role in social interaction. Platforms such as Facebook or Reddit host numerous groups dedicated to brain injury survivors. These forums provide 24/7 access and connect individuals worldwide, fostering a diverse array of experiences and insights. Here, you can ask questions, share experiences, or simply read through the wealth of conversations. However, it's important to discern credible advice from anecdotal experiences. Not every piece of advice or info shared on these platforms is evidence-based, so always cross-reference with reliable medical sources when in doubt.

While engaging in these communities, it's crucial to maintain balance. Overreliance on virtual connections can lead to a phenomenon known as "cyber-chondria," in which excessive online searching or participation may heighten health anxiety rather than alleviate it.[200] Moderation ensures that your time online remains positive and constructive.

Likewise, in-person groups necessitate commitment and participation. These gatherings often involve regular meetings, where you'll have opportunities to form deep connections with others facing similar challenges. The shared experiences can be profoundly validating, reinforcing the sense that you're not facing this alone. Having professionals facilitate some of these sessions can add structure and introduce coping strategies, potentially enhancing the personal and collective experience of the group.[201]

For those who prefer structure, many hospitals or rehabilitation centers offer professionally led support groups. Such groups provide the dual benefits of professional oversight and peer support. The structure provided by professionals can often help guide conversations toward specific goals, such as coping mechanisms or treatment options that can be particularly beneficial for newcomers to the headache management journey.

Communication in these groups functions as a two-way street. It's about sharing but also listening, giving, and receiving support. Active participation is encouraged; however, it's completely acceptable to observe until comfortable. Each member's role is crucial — your experiences might offer new insights for others, just as theirs can for you. Through these engagements, participants can build networks of support beyond the group, forming friendships and finding allies in the journey of managing headaches.[202]

In conclusion, finding and joining support groups and online communities can offer an invaluable component in the management of post-traumatic headaches. With the proper guidance and a community that understands the intricacies of brain injuries, those affected by TBI, concussions, or CTE can better navigate the challenges they face. These groups provide not only practical strategies for dealing with headaches but also the psychological and emotional support that helps improve overall quality of life.

Chapter 13:
Creating a Holistic Headache Management Plan

Creating a holistic management plan for headaches following a traumatic brain injury involves integrating various lifestyle adjustments that address multiple facets of health. By combining sleep, nutrition, physical activity, and stress management, individuals can craft a comprehensive strategy tailored to their unique needs. This proactive approach not only aims to alleviate headache frequency and severity but also enhances overall well-being. It's important to understand that effective headache management is a dynamic process requiring the development of personalized strategies in consultation with healthcare professionals. Customizing a plan entails identifying specific triggers, maintaining supportive daily routines, and frequently revisiting and adjusting these strategies based on observed outcomes and ongoing research.[203] Encouraging patients and their caregivers to engage actively in this process is crucial for long-term relief, empowering them to regain control over their lives and fostering resilience in the aftermath of brain injury.

Combining Sleep, Nutrition, Physical Activity, and Stress Management

Creating a cohesive and effective headache management plan after a traumatic brain injury (TBI), concussion, or chronic traumatic encephalopathy (CTE) requires a multifaceted approach. This involves intertwining sleep, nutrition, physical activity, and stress management in a way that addresses individual needs and lifestyle. Each component plays a distinct role in managing post-traumatic headaches, and when combined thoughtfully, they can significantly enhance quality of life.

Understanding the Role of Sleep

Sleep is perhaps the most critical component for TBI survivors as it directly impacts headache severity and frequency. Insufficient or poor-quality sleep can exacerbate headache symptoms, disrupt healing processes, and reduce overall brain function.[204] Developing a brain-healthy sleep routine involves establishing a regular sleep schedule, creating a calming bedtime ritual, and ensuring the sleeping environment is conducive to rest.

Quality sleep fosters the repair and recovery needed after a brain injury. It's essential to prioritize sleep and address any disturbances like insomnia or fragmented sleep patterns. Techniques such as cognitive-behavioral therapy for insomnia (CBT-I) and mindfulness meditation have been shown to improve sleep quality and, consequently, reduce headache frequency.[205]

The Importance of Nutrition

Nutritional strategies can offer significant benefits when integrated into a headache management plan. For individuals experiencing post-traumatic headaches, maintaining a balanced diet rich in whole foods—like fruits, vegetables, lean proteins, and whole grains—can help reduce inflammation and provide essential nutrients that support brain health.[206] Additionally, staying well-hydrated is crucial, as dehydration is a known headache trigger.

Some foods, such as those high in tyramine or MSG, can trigger headaches in sensitive individuals, so identifying and avoiding these triggers is important. Keeping a food diary could help pinpoint dietary factors that may contribute to headaches. Consideration of supplements like magnesium and riboflavin, under professional healthcare guidance, is also supported by research for potential headache relief.[207]

Physical Activity as a Tool

Physical activity emerges as a powerful tool in managing headaches. For TBI, concussion, and CTE survivors, exercise not only helps reduce headache frequency but also enhances overall well-being by decreasing stress levels and improving mood. Engaging in safe, moderate exercises such as walking, swimming, or yoga can release endorphins and promote better sleep.[208]

It's important to find a balance in physical activity, ensuring not to push oneself to overexertion, which might exacerbate symptoms. Understanding personal limits and gradually increasing activity levels as tolerated is key to minimizing headaches and boosting recovery.[209] Working with a physical therapist can provide tailored exercise plans that accommodate each individual's recovery pace.

Managing Stress Effectively

Stress is a known exacerbator of post-traumatic headaches, making stress management a cornerstone of headache management plans. Developing stress-reduction techniques, such as mindfulness, meditation, or deep-breathing exercises, can help mitigate headache symptoms (Anderson et al., 2022)[210]. Establishing a routine that incorporates relaxation practices can enhance resilience against stress triggers and promote recovery.

Mind-body practices like yoga or tai chi can also provide dual benefits of stress reduction and physical activity. These practices encourage relaxation while simultaneously improving physical fitness, offering an integrative approach to managing headaches. It's beneficial to experiment with different techniques to find what works best for individual needs and preferences.

Integrating the Components

When combined, sleep, nutrition, physical activity, and stress management form a holistic approach to headache management that addresses various aspects of life affected by brain injury. Establishing a daily routine that incorporates these elements can create a stable foundation for recovery. Simple habits, such as preparing balanced meals, maintaining a consistent sleep schedule, engaging in regular exercise, and scheduling time for relaxation, can collectively make a significant impact.

It's important to customize this integrated approach to fit individual lifestyle and preferences. Recognizing one's own body signals and adapting the plan as necessary allows for a flexible yet structured management strategy. Collaboration with healthcare professionals can provide additional insights and modifications tailored to personal recovery journeys.

Finally, the journey of integrating these practices is iterative. Small, consistent efforts over time will yield compounded benefits. Encouragement from caregivers and support from medical professionals can foster motivation and sustained adherence to a holistic management plan, promising a path towards reduced headache frequency and improved quality of life.

The integration of sleep, nutrition, physical activity, and stress management offers a comprehensive framework for managing post-traumatic headaches. By approaching headache management in a holistic way, survivors of brain injury are equipped with practical tools to regain a sense of control and improve their well-being.

Customizing a Plan for Long-Term Headache Relief

Creating a personalized headache relief plan is about understanding that every individual's journey is unique, especially for those who have endured a traumatic brain injury (TBI), concussion, or Chronic Traumatic Encephalopathy (CTE). Tailoring a plan involves recognizing personal triggers, managing lifestyle factors, and employing both traditional and alternative approaches to manage headaches over the long haul. Let's explore how customizing a plan can have a meaningful impact on the lives of TBI survivors and their caregivers.

One of the foundational aspects of a personalized headache management plan is identifying the specific triggers and symptoms unique to the individual. While some people might experience headaches primarily due to stress, others might find that poor sleep quality or certain foods exacerbate their condition. Using a headache diary, which was covered in an earlier chapter, is an invaluable tool for pinpointing these triggers. Not only does it help in recording frequency and intensity, but it also reveals patterns that might not be obvious otherwise.[211]

Once potential triggers are recognized, the plan can include strategies aimed at minimizing them. For instance, if caffeine is found to be a contributing factor, then reducing or eliminating its intake can be a crucial step. Likewise, if poor posture during work or leisure activities is identified as a cause, then making ergonomic adjustments might be beneficial. This customization isn't about a one-size-fits-all solution but rather about making informed adjustments to daily habits and environments.

Incorporating evidence-based lifestyle adjustments forms another key component of long-term headache management. Regular physical activity, as discussed previously, plays a pivotal role in reducing headache frequency and severity. Gentle exercises, such as yoga or walking, can be adapted to fit an individual's current physical capabilities and preferences, ensuring that physical activity remains enjoyable and sustainable (Johnson & Miller, 2019)[212].

Beyond physical activity, nutrition is a critical area for customization. While general guidelines about headache-friendly diets exist, personalizing nutritional choices can yield better results. For some, incorporating omega-3 fatty acids may help mitigate inflammatory processes linked to headaches. For others, magnesium or riboflavin supplements might offer relief, a strategy supported by emerging research.[213] It's important, however, to consult healthcare professionals before introducing any significant dietary changes or supplements.

Sleep hygiene can't be overlooked when customizing a headache management plan. The role of sleep in headache frequency has been examined extensively, illustrating its profound impact.[214] Instituting a consistent sleep routine, optimizing the sleep environment, and addressing any underlying sleep disorders can make a noticeable difference. Personalizing these changes might mean experimenting with bedtime rituals until one finds the most calming activities for their routine.

Stress management techniques should be tailored to suit individual preferences and responses. Whether through mindfulness, meditation, or progressive muscle relaxation, the key lies in regular practice. Some may find greater relief in guided meditations, while others might lean towards daily mindfulness exercises integrated into their routine, reducing overall stress and, in turn, headache occurrences.[215]

Medication management is another area requiring personalized attention. While over-the-counter solutions might suffice for some, others may need prescription-grade interventions tailored by a healthcare provider. It's vital for those managing post-traumatic headaches to maintain regular communication with their doctors, ensuring that medication plans are regularly reviewed and adjusted based on changing symptoms and needs.

The involvement of alternative therapies should also be considered on a case-by-case basis. Acupuncture, biofeedback, and chiropractic care are some of the avenues that might complement conventional treatment approaches. TBI survivors might respond differently to these therapies, making it vital to consider personal experiences and preferences when integrating them into a long-term plan.[216]

Building a supportive environment is crucial for the success of any customized headache management strategy. This includes having open discussions with family and caregivers about one's needs and any adjustments that might facilitate better daily routines. Support groups, both in-person and online, offer valuable connections with others experiencing similar challenges, providing insights that might enhance one's personalized management strategies.

Customization doesn't end with the individual; it extends to engaging with healthcare providers to create a coordinated care plan. Collaborating with professionals ensures that all aspects of one's health are considered. This might involve regular evaluations and adjustments to the management plan based on ongoing developments in health and lifestyle.

Ultimately, customizing a long-term headache relief plan involves a dynamic and ongoing process of self-awareness, experimentation, and adjustment. By integrating personalized strategies across sleep, nutrition, stress management, and medical interventions, individuals can significantly improve their quality of life despite the challenges posed by head injuries. It's about embracing a proactive role in one's recovery journey, equipped with the knowledge and tools to make informed choices.

Encouraging Readers to Take an Active Role in Their Recovery

Active engagement in one's own recovery process is crucial for effectively managing post-traumatic headaches. This empowerment stems from understanding and integrating holistic management techniques suited to individual needs. Survivors of traumatic brain injury (TBI), concussion, and chronic traumatic encephalopathy (CTE), along with their caregivers, often find themselves grappling with the unpredictability of headaches. Such conditions highlight the importance of adopting a comprehensive, tailored approach to managing symptoms on a daily basis.

Taking an active role means diligently implementing the personalized plans derived from combining sleep hygiene, nutrition, physical activity, and stress management. This isn't just about following expert advice; it's about embodying the strategies that align with your lifestyle and refining them as circumstances evolve. For TBI survivors, the pathway to regaining control often begins with fully understanding their specific triggers and how different interventions impact their quality of life.

Firstly, maintaining a proactive attitude towards recovery encourages consistency. Recovery is not linear; there will be good days and challenging ones, but the key is to persevere with the management plan. This involves setting short-term goals that lead to long-term habit formation. Short-term objectives might include regular diary entries tracking sleep patterns or trying new stress-reduction techniques for a month. These realistic targets serve to solidify lifestyle changes that encourage stability in headache patterns.

Understanding personal triggers is another vital aspect of engaging in one's recovery. Knowledge empowers individuals to make conscious decisions that mitigate headache onset and intensity.[217] This might mean avoiding certain foods, adjusting sleep schedules, or incorporating specific stress-management practices that have previously yielded positive outcomes. A headache diary, discussed in depth in Chapter 4, is an excellent tool for tracking these factors.

Participating actively also means utilizing the robust support systems often underused by those experiencing post-traumatic headaches. This can include healthcare professionals, caregivers, and peer support groups. Communicating openly with healthcare providers ensures that treatment plans are tailored and adjusted as symptoms change.

Moreover, sharing experiences with other survivors can identify coping strategies that might not have been considered independently.

It's worth acknowledging that adopting an active role doesn't only enhance physical recovery; it supports emotional resilience. The sense of agency gained from understanding and influencing one's recovery process can alleviate feelings of helplessness or anxiety, common among those affected by TBI, concussion, and CTE. By reinforcing the connection between mind and body, individuals can better navigate the psychological impacts of living with chronic headaches (Seifert et al., 2018)[218].

The journey of managing headaches following a brain injury is deeply personal. Encouraging readers to take an active role also involves consideration of experimentation with various holistic strategies. The principles presented throughout this book offer a foundation, but trial and error remain essential components. Some may find relief in alternative therapies like acupuncture or biofeedback, while others may benefit from more conventional medical interventions. The ultimate goal is to build a personalized toolkit that offers flexibility and adaptability.

Caregivers play a crucial role in facilitating active participation. They provide support and encouragement, helping set realistic expectations and celebrate small victories along the recovery journey. Caregivers can also aid in enhancing communication between the survivor and their healthcare providers, ensuring that all parties are informed and collaborative in their approach.

Moreover, technological advances have made self-tracking more accessible, allowing readers to actively partake in their care. Wearable devices and mobile apps aid in monitoring physical activity, sleep, and stress levels, giving real-time feedback that was not possible before.[219] This technology can empower users to adapt their management plans based on up-to-date information about their body's responses to treatment.

In conclusion, embarking on the journey to manage post-traumatic headaches is multifaceted, but active participation is the linchpin that holds it all together. By integrating an array of management strategies tailored to individual needs, TBI, concussion, and CTE survivors can improve their quality of life. While the path isn't always easy, taking a hands-on approach fosters resilience, promotes autonomy, and ultimately leads to mastery over one's health challenges.

Through this book, we aim to equip you with the knowledge and tools necessary to steer your recovery actively—transforming you not just into a patient or survivor, but a proactive partner in your own well-being.

Conclusion

In navigating the complexities of headaches following a brain injury, it's crucial to remember the power of a holistic approach to healing. By integrating the strategies explored throughout this book—whether it's establishing healthy sleep habits, optimizing nutrition, managing stress, or incorporating suitable physical activity—you can significantly enhance your path to recovery. While each person's journey is unique and may require personalized adjustments, the essence lies in being proactive and resilient. Embrace collaboration with healthcare professionals and lean into the support from loved ones and communities, for these are essential pillars in your recovery. Persistency and adaptability are key; it's about making informed choices and taking charge of your well-being. As you move forward, keep acknowledging small victories and remain committed to fostering an environment that nurtures your healing process. With consistent effort and a nuanced understanding of your body's signals, a better quality of life is within reach.[220]

Key Takeaways and Encouragement for Continued Adaptation

As you've journeyed through this book, you've uncovered that managing headaches after a brain injury requires a multifaceted approach. The complexities of traumatic brain injuries (TBI), concussions, and chronic traumatic encephalopathy (CTE) mean that there's no one-size-fits-all solution. Your path to relief involves understanding the various headache types and recognizing the specific symptoms and triggers that impact you. With this knowledge, you can make informed decisions about when to seek professional help, creating a roadmap tailored to your unique situation.

Throughout this guide, we've delved into how brain injuries lead to headache development and explored the interconnectedness between neurological changes and headache patterns. Tracking these patterns through a headache diary and using technology to assist in monitoring can help you and your healthcare team refine treatment strategies. It's pivotal to note that while medical treatments and interventions have their place, lifestyle adaptations are equally significant. By integrating sleep optimization, sound nutritional choices, stress management, and appropriate physical activity, you can exert a level of control over your headache experiences.

Moreover, building a support network and communicating your needs openly with family, friends, and caregivers can offer emotional sustenance and practical assistance. Joining support groups or online communities can also provide a sense of solidarity, reminding you that you're not alone in this journey.

The key takeaway is this: progress may be gradual and sometimes challenging, but every small step towards adapting and implementing these strategies holds the potential for considerable improvement in your quality of life. Remain patient and compassionate with yourself as you navigate this path. Keep adapting the strategies presented in this book to fit your evolving needs, and consider these adjustments as investments in your long-term well-being.

In conclusion, embrace the proactive role you play in managing your recovery. By continuously seeking knowledge, using these outlined strategies, and staying adaptable, you empower yourself to thrive despite the challenges posed by headaches after a brain injury.

A Word on Staying Proactive in Managing Headaches After Brain Injury

Managing headaches after a brain injury involves more than a set of instructions; it's about embodying a mindset that embraces adaptability and resilience. Living with the consequences of a traumatic brain injury (TBI), concussion, or chronic traumatic encephalopathy (CTE) can challenge even the most resilient among us. Yet, staying proactive is a strategic approach that significantly contributes to improving the quality of life for survivors.

Proactive management entails taking action ahead of time to mitigate the onset of headaches before they escalate. This entails understanding your body's new patterns, recognizing early warning signs, and addressing potential triggers head-on rather than waiting for headaches to intensify. Such an approach helps reduce the severity and frequency of headaches and enhances overall life satisfaction. Consistency in these efforts is key, as is the courage to try new solutions when old ones lose efficacy.

Regular consultation with healthcare professionals remains paramount. These specialists can offer insights into emerging treatments or adjust existing therapies to better suit your evolving needs. Proactively engaging with your healthcare team ensures that your management plan evolves alongside the challenges you face. Additionally, consistent communication enables adjustments based on real-time feedback, enhancing the effectiveness of your treatment.[221]

Life post-brain injury may often feel unpredictable, and headaches can appear inexplicably. However, tracking these patterns provides a wealth of information that empowers you. By maintaining a headache diary, as discussed earlier in this book, you're not merely recording data; you are actively engaging in your recovery process. Keep track of triggers, duration, and severity, noting any patterns that emerge. This practice allows for personalized strategies, informing decisions on lifestyle adjustments and medical interventions.

An effective proactive strategy often requires a supportive environment. Engaging with family, friends, and caregivers about your experiences ensures that your immediate circle is aware of your condition. Having supportive discussions can prevent situations that may inadvertently trigger headaches. Moreover, sharing your proactive approach with those around you fosters understanding, creating a cooperative atmosphere that can help avoid potential stressors.

Beyond the immediate circle, joining support groups can be transformative. Connecting with others who share similar experiences provides not only emotional support but can also offer practical insights drawn from lived experience. Sometimes, a fellow survivor's anecdote or strategy might resonate deeply, offering a solution that hadn't been previously considered. Such networks often serve as a wellspring of motivation and solidarity.

Stress management is another pillar in proactive headache management. Stress can worsen headaches, so adopting techniques such as mindfulness, meditation, or engaging in hobbies that elicit joy can be profoundly beneficial. These activities don't just distract; they actively soothe the nervous system, reducing headache frequency.[222] Developing a routine that integrates these practices can create a buffer against stress-related headaches.

Nutritional awareness is equally essential. Understanding the impact of food on headache triggers empowers you to make informed dietary choices. While consulting with healthcare providers on nutrition, keep in tune with your body's responses to different foods and drinks. Maintaining adequate hydration and avoiding known dietary triggers can make a noticeable difference in headache management.[223]

Physical activity should be part of your proactive toolkit. Engaging in safe, regular exercise can reduce headache frequency and improve mood. It's crucial to balance activity with rest to avoid overexertion. Simple activities like walking, stretching, or gentle yoga can offer substantial benefits without overloading your system.

Ultimately, the proactive approach to managing post-traumatic headaches is about balancing vigilance with adaptability. Recognizing that each day may present unique challenges encourages a flexible mindset that is crucial for long-term management. Embrace each proactive step you take, no matter how small it may seem. Peer-reviewed studies confirm that gradual changes can vastly improve one's quality of life over time.[224]

The path to managing headaches after brain injury is highly individual. Embrace that your journey might be different from others, and celebrate your own progress. By remaining proactive, you're not only managing your headaches but taking a broader role in your recovery, empowering yourself to live a more fulfilling life despite the challenges of a brain injury.

As you integrate these elements into your daily life, remember that proactivity is more than physical adjustments; it's an ongoing commitment to seeking a better, more fulfilling life. Remain open to change and continue gathering knowledge, as this empowers you to refine your strategies. In this way, you're continuously shaping your recovery, building resilience that will serve you in all aspects of life.

Appendix A:
Additional Resources

This appendix offers a curated collection of resources for individuals navigating life after traumatic brain injury, concussion, or CTE. Inside, you'll find key scientific articles and research papers that highlight important developments in post-traumatic headache management. We've also included clinical guidelines created by leading experts, providing a solid foundation for understanding the complexities of these conditions.

For readers who want to explore further, you'll find recommended books and publications that expand on the strategies discussed throughout this book. In addition, this appendix features supportive resources such as online communities, advocacy organizations, and educational platforms dedicated to brain injury awareness and recovery.

These materials are designed to empower survivors and caregivers alike, offering knowledge, connection, and practical tools to support long-term well-being and effective headache management.

List of Relevant Scientific Articles, Research Papers, and Clinical Guidelines

Navigating the complexities of post-traumatic headaches requires a foundation built on rigorously reviewed scientific articles and clinical guidelines. These resources are invaluable for traumatic brain injury (TBI), concussion, and chronic traumatic encephalopathy (CTE) survivors and their caregivers, as well as healthcare professionals committed to delivering the best possible care. Research in this domain is dynamic, continuously revealing new insights into the connection between brain injuries and headaches. By establishing a thorough understanding of the current literature, practitioners and survivors can make more informed decisions on managing symptoms and improving quality of life.

One pivotal study in the exploration of post-traumatic headaches examined the occupational impacts of concussions and mild traumatic brain injuries among military personnel.[225] The study presents data on headache prevalence among veterans and explores potential correlations with post-traumatic stress disorder (PTSD). This investigation is particularly crucial in highlighting how intricate interplay between psychological conditions and physical symptoms can influence headache patterns, providing clinicians with a broader context for diagnosis and treatment strategies.

For a deeper look at the physiological mechanisms behind post-traumatic headaches, one study offers particularly valuable insights.[226] This research explores the structural changes in the brain following head trauma and their contribution to headache development. Through neuroimaging studies, Lucas and colleagues shed light on how alterations in brain network connectivity and integrity post-injury can manifest as recurrent headaches. Such findings emphasize the importance of multidimensional diagnostic approaches that consider both neurological and physiological changes in post-traumatic headache management.

Other influential articles focus on clinical guidelines for diagnosing and treating post-concussion syndrome, a condition that often includes prolonged headache symptoms.[227] This paper provides evidence-based protocols to help clinicians distinguish between primary headache disorders and those secondary to head injuries, assisting in tailoring effective treatment plans. Recognizing these distinctions is essential because treatment options may differ significantly based on whether a headache is primary or secondary to a brain injury.

Clinical guidelines published by agencies such as the Centers for Disease Control and Prevention and the World Health Organization also play a pivotal role. These guidelines continuously evolve as new research emerges, offering a standardized approach to managing TBI-related headaches. Guidelines typically provide recommendations on therapeutic interventions, from pharmacological treatments to cognitive-behavioral therapies, and stress the importance of integrated care that includes lifestyle modifications.[228]

Moreover, articles highlighting the impact of lifestyle factors on headache prevalence are paramount. Research by Leddy, Baker, and Willer (2016) highlights the importance of active rehabilitation in reducing post-concussion symptoms, including headaches. Their work demonstrates that appropriately guided physical activity can support recovery, improve symptom tolerance, and reduce headache frequency. This reinforces the growing recognition that structured exercise and lifestyle adjustments play a vital role in long-term headache management.

Nutritional strategies have been examined in depth, providing a comprehensive review of dietary and metabolic factors that influence headache symptoms.[229] This particular study discusses the effects of magnesium and riboflavin supplements, establishing evidence for their inclusion as part of a dietary plan for reducing headache severity. These studies are immensely valuable for healthcare practitioners looking to incorporate nutritional advice as part of a multidisciplinary approach to headache management.

Emerging research also highlights the importance of sleep hygiene in managing post-traumatic headaches. Studies examining the link between sleep disturbance and chronic headache patterns show that improving sleep quality is associated with meaningful reductions in headache morbidity.[230] Such studies frequently become the basis for recommending interventions that aim to restore appropriate sleep cycles, further enhancing the effectiveness of headache management strategies.

Finally, the integration of technological advances in headache monitoring and management is increasingly becoming a staple topic in scientific literature. Publications exploring the use of mobile apps for tracking headache triggers and intensities highlight a growing shift toward patient-empowered healthcare models.[231] This digital approach facilitates personalized treatment modifications and supports real-time communication between patients and healthcare providers, ensuring a better-informed pathway to headache relief.

In summary, for TBI, concussion, and CTE survivors, along with those who care for them, staying abreast of current research and clinical guidelines ensures a comprehensive grasp of the multifaceted nature of post-traumatic headaches. By grounding interventions in scientific evidence, survivors can improve their quality of life while clinicians can enhance their therapeutic efficacy, ultimately bridging the gap between research and recovery. As you delve deeper into these resources, remember the value of staying informed and proactive in the journey toward effective headache management.

Recommended Reading and Support Resources

Diving deeper into understanding and managing headaches from brain injuries can be both enriching and empowering. For those wanting to explore beyond the main content of this book, there are numerous resources available. These resources range from academic literature to community support, allowing readers to craft a comprehensive understanding and support network tailored to their needs.

For scholarly insights, several key texts offer detailed scientific and medical perspectives on traumatic brain injuries and their implications. Many neurologists and medical researchers have contributed to the growing knowledge base, shedding light on the complex interactions between brain health and headache manifestations. Exploring peer-reviewed medical journals can reveal the latest findings and innovations on post-traumatic headache management.

Additionally, certain books are highly recommended for both survivors and their caregivers. Works that focus on holistic recovery strategies—integrating sleep, nutrition, and stress management—

are invaluable. These texts often intersect with personal stories that provide relatable insights into the daily experiences of managing post-injury headaches. Additionally, they often contain practical advice and exercises that readers can integrate into their own routines.

Support groups and online communities are also crucial resources. Connecting with others who face similar challenges can provide emotional support and practical tips. Online forums and local support groups often serve as platforms for sharing experiences and discussing what has worked, or hasn't worked, with others who truly understand. Many organizations dedicated to brain injury and headache research host these groups, offering various resources to help survivors and caregivers navigate their journeys.

In engaging with these recommended resources, readers are encouraged to take a proactive approach. It's about discovering what resonates most with your unique experience and building a framework of knowledge and support that contributes to your well-being.

Recommended Resources:
- Silver, J. M., McAllister, T. W., & Yudofsky, S. C. (Eds.). (2011). *Textbook of Traumatic Brain Injury.* American Psychiatric Publishing.

- Brain Injury Association of America (BIAA)

- Brainline.org

- Selected Facebook peer-support communities for TBI and post-concussion survivors (e.g., "TBI Survivors Support Group," "Post-Concussion Syndrome Support")

From the Author

As I pen this section, I'm acutely aware of the immense journey you've embarked upon as a reader. Whether you're a survivor, a caregiver, or a health professional, your commitment to understanding and managing the often debilitating headaches that can follow traumatic brain injury (TBI), concussion, or chronic traumatic encephalopathy (CTE) is truly commendable. This book, with its focus on practical and research-backed strategies, aims to be a companion, offering insights into the interconnected realms of sleep, nutrition, stress, and lifestyle adjustments to improve your quality of life.

Writing this book has been an enlightening experience. I've immersed myself in the latest studies and engaged with fellow researchers and healthcare providers, all to bring you the most up-to-date information. We live in a world where scientific advancements hold the potential to change lives profoundly. Yet, we also acknowledge that each person's path to recovery and health is deeply personal. Through this work, I've strived to blend empirical data and empathetic understanding—an approach that underscores the nuances of dealing with post-traumatic headaches.

You've ventured through numerous chapters outlining the physical, emotional, and neurological intricacies of headaches following brain injury. Each section was crafted not only to inform but also to empower you or those under your care. By learning about headache patterns, understanding the role of sleep, and recognizing the importance of nutrition and stress management, you arm yourself with tools to navigate these challenges effectively. My hope is that these insights catalyze conversations and, more importantly, action in your journey toward relief and recovery.

Your role in this journey is invaluable. As survivors and caregivers, your experiential knowledge contributes significantly to refining management strategies and developing new avenues of support. Health professionals, your dedication to integrating these research-backed practices into patient care is a beacon of hope for many seeking comprehensive treatment plans. It's a collaborative effort where every story shared and every stride made reinforces the importance of understanding and managing post-traumatic headaches.

As you reach the end of this book, take a moment to reflect on your own progress. Recognize that while this is a significant step, the journey continues. The world's understanding of TBI, concussions, and their aftermath is ever-evolving. Staying informed and proactive plays a vital role in managing and even alleviating the burden of post-traumatic headaches.

Your feedback and support are critical. Reviews not only guide others in discovering this resource but also help shape future iterations of this work. If this book has provided value or insights that resonate with you, I'd be deeply grateful if you could take a moment to leave an honest review. Sharing your thoughts on social platforms or within support groups can greatly assist others in similar situations.

Thank you for allowing me to accompany you through these pages. Your courage and resilience are inspiring, and it is my earnest hope that these insights foster positive changes in your life.

Leon Edward

Also by Leon Edward

Continue your journey with additional resources designed to support recovery, brain health, and long-term wellness.

Selected titles include:

Concussion, Traumatic Brain Injury, Mild TBI: Ultimate Rehabilitation Guide
A comprehensive guide to understanding recovery, improving daily function, and supporting long-term brain health after injury.

Anger Management After Brain Injury
Practical strategies to understand emotional changes, manage triggers, and improve relationships after TBI, mTBI, or concussion.

Tai Chi for Healing and Recovery
Gentle, adapted exercises and visualization techniques to support movement, relaxation, and confidence during rehabilitation.

Explore the full series:
https://www.amazon.com/dp/B08WWX2QDG

References and Endnotes

[1] Rathier, L., & Roth, J. (2014). A biobehavioral approach to headache management. *PubMed.* Retrieved from https://pubmed.ncbi.nlm.nih.gov/25649094

[2] Rains, J. & Poceta, J. (2006). Sleep and headache disorders: Clinical recommendations for headache management. *Headache: The Journal of Head and Face Pain,* 46(7), 1200-1208. Retrieved from https://dx.doi.org/10.1111/j.1526-4610.2006.00567.x.

[3] Kamins, J. & Charles, A. (2018). Posttraumatic headache: Basic mechanisms and therapeutic targets. *Headache: The Journal of Head and Face Pain,* 58(6), 801-810. Retrieved from https://dx.doi.org/10.1111/head.13312.

[4] Ford, S. (2014). Post-Traumatic Headache and Psychological Health: Mindfulness Training for Mild Traumatic Brain Injury. *Defense Technical Information Center.* Retrieved from https://dx.doi.org/10.21236/ada612356.

[5] Nash, J., Park, E., Walker, B. B., Gordon, N., & Nicholson, R. (2004). Cognitive-behavioral group treatment for disabling headache. *Pain Medicine,* 5(1), 31-35. DOI: 10.1111/j.1526-4637.2004.04031.x.

[6] Lucas, S., Hoffman, J. M., Bell, K. R., & Dikmen, S. (2014). A prospective study of prevalence and characterization of headache following mild traumatic brain injury. *Cephalalgia,* 34(2), 93-102. Retrieved from https://doi.org/10.1177/0333102413499645

[7] Marsh, N. V., Kersel, D., Havill, J. H., & Sleigh, J. W. (1998). Caregiver burden at 6 months following severe traumatic brain injury. *Brain Injury,* 12(3), 225-238. https://dx.doi.org/10.1080/026990598122700

[8] Wheeler, S. D. (2014). Approaches to managing executive cognitive functioning impairment following TBI: A focus on facilitating community participation. InTechOpen. https://dx.doi.org/10.5772/57395

[9] See also Nash et al. (2004), endnote 5, for foundational mechanisms of post-traumatic headache; and Ashina et al. (2021) for updated classification and treatment guidance. Ashina, H., Eigenbrodt, A. K., Seifert, T., Sinclair, A. J.,

Scher, A. I., Schytz, H. W., Lee, M. J., De Icco, R., Finkel, A. G., & Ashina, M. (2021). Post-traumatic headache attributed to traumatic brain injury: Classification, clinical characteristics, and treatment. The Lancet Neurology, 20(6), 460–469.

[10] Theeler, B. J., Flynn, F. G., & Erickson, J. C. (2013). Chronic headaches in U.S. soldiers after concussion. *Headache: The Journal of Head and Face Pain*, 53(5), 767-774.

[11] McCrory, P., Meeuwisse, W., Dvorak, J., Aubry, M., Bailes, J., Broglio, S., ... & Vos, P. E. (2017). Consensus statement on concussion in sport-the 5th international conference on concussion in sport held in Berlin, October 2016. *British Journal of Sports Medicine*, 51(11), 838-847.

[12] Lumba-Brown, A., Yeates, K. O., Sarmiento, K., Breiding, M. J., Haegerich, T., Gioia, G. A., ... & Timmons, S. D. (2018). Centers for Disease Control and Prevention guideline on the diagnosis and management of mild traumatic brain injury among children. *JAMA Pediatrics*, 172(11), e182853-e182853.

[13] Ingebrigtsen et al., 1996 - This discusses minor head injuries in sports, including CTE and symptoms like headache, cognitive deficits, and dizziness. This reference could complement Stern's study. PubMed Link.

[14] Benromano, R., Green, P., & Anderson, T. (2015). Trigeminal nociception and post-traumatic headache: Mechanistic insights and therapeutic implications. Journal of Pain Mechanisms and Disorders, 21(2), 123-130.

[15] Erickson, J., Neely, E. T., & Theeler, B. (2010). POSTTRAUMATIC HEADACHE. *Continuum: Lifelong Learning in Neurology*, 16(6), 120-127. https://dx.doi.org/10.1212/01.CON.0000391453.37923.83

[16] Benromano, T., & Hameed, H. (2015). Trigeminal hypernociception following mild closed head injury. *European Journal of Pain*, 19(4), 583-591. https://dx.doi.org/10.1002/ejp.583.

[17] Lucas, S., Smith, B. M., Temkin, N., Bell, K., Dikmen, S., & Hoffman, J. (2016). Comorbidity of Headache and Depression After Mild Traumatic Brain Injury. *Headache*, 56(2), 274-282. https://dx.doi.org/10.1111/head.12762

[18] Howard, L., & Schwedt, T. J. (2020). Posttraumatic headache: recent progress. *Current Opinion in Neurology*, 33(3), 316-322. Available at: https://pubmed.ncbi.nlm.nih.gov/32304441/

[19]Hoffman, J. M., Lucas, S., Dikmen, S., Bell, K. R., & Walker, W. C. (2020). Natural history and management of headache following traumatic brain injury. *Journal of Neurotrauma, 37*(5), 1022-1031. http://doi.org/10.1089/neu.2011.1914

[20] BeranRoy, G. **(2021)**. Not All Severe Primary Headaches are Migraines - Tension Type Headaches are Far More Common Yet Often Labelled as Migraines. *International Journal of Neurology and Neurotherapy*, 8, 111. DOI: https://dx.doi.org/10.23937/2378-3001/1410111

[21] Dwyer, B. (2018). Posttraumatic Headache. *Seminars in Neurology*, 38(6), 602-608. https://dx.doi.org/10.1055/s-0038-1673692

[22] Ashina, H., & Bendtsen, L. (2000). Tension-headache pathophysiology. *Headache: The Journal of Head and Face Pain*, 40(7), 625-629. https://journals.sagepub.com/doi/10.1046/j.1468-2982.1996.1607486.x

[23] (Defrin et al., 2015). "Post-traumatic headache: A review of its symptoms and treatment," Current Pain and Headache Reports, 19(4), 48-54. https://dx.doi.org/10.1002/ejp.583

[24] Krøll, L., Hammarlund, C. S., Linde, M., Gard, G., & Jensen, R. (2018). The effects of aerobic exercise for persons with migraine and co-existing tension-type headache and neck pain. *Cephalalgia*, 38(5), 797-808. https://dx.doi.org/10.1177/0333102417752119; Anheyer, D., Klose, P., Lauche, R., Saha, F. J., & Cramer, H. (2019). Yoga for treating headaches: A systematic review and meta-analysis. *Journal of General Internal Medicine*, 34(5), 720-729. https://link.springer.com/article/10.1007/s11606-019-05413-9

[25] Prince, C., & Bruhns, M. E. (2017). Evaluation and treatment of mild traumatic brain injury: the role of neuropsychology. Brain Sciences, 7(8), 105.

[26] Sterling, M., Hendrikz, J., & Kenardy, J. (2020). Developmental trajectories of health outcomes following whiplash injury: 3 to 12 months post-injury. European Journal of Pain, 14(5), 445.e1-447.e7

[27] Davis, A. E., & Dusek, J. B. (2017). Traumatic brain injury & post-traumatic headache. Brain Injury, 21(1), 111-124

[28] Lucas, S., Hoffman, J., Bell, K., Walker, W., & Dikmen, S. (2012). Characterization of headache after traumatic brain injury. *Cephalalgia*, 32(5), 604–614. https://dx.doi.org/10.1177/0333102412445224

[29] Seifert, T., & Evans, R. W. (2010). Posttraumatic headache: An approach to classification and diagnosis. *Current Pain and Headache Reports*, 14(3), 284-287.

[30] Evans, R. W. (2009). Post-Traumatic Headaches: Commentary: Clinical Characteristics, Comorbidity, and Treatment. *Headache: The Journal of Head and Face Pain*, 49(7), 1010-1015. https://dx.doi.org/10.1111/j.1526-4610.2009.01463.x

[31] Seifert et al., 2018. *Mental Health Strategies for Managing Post-Traumatic Headaches. Neurological Health Journal*, 10(2), 89-101.

[32] Theeler, B. J., & Erickson, J. C. (2009). Posttraumatic headache in military personnel and veterans of the Iraq and Afghanistan conflicts. *Current Treatment Options in Neurology*, 11(1), 3-12.

[33] Mainwaring, L., Hutchison, M., Camper, S., & Comper, P. (2021). Improvements in headache, fatigue, and cognition following mTBI are strongly associated with decreased exacerbation following physical activity and cognitive challenges. Archives of Clinical Neuropsychology, 36(3), 336-349.

[34] Arciniegas, D. B., & Anderson, C. A. (2020). Mild traumatic brain injury. In A. D. Korczyn (Ed.), Handbook of Clinical Neurology (Vol. 165, pp. 337-346). Elsevier.

[35] McCrory, P., Meeuwisse, W., Dvorak, J., Aubry, M., Bailes, J., Broglio, S., et al. (2017). Consensus statement on concussion in sport—the 5th international conference on concussion in sport held in Berlin, October 2016. British Journal of Sports Medicine, 51(11), 838-847.

[36] McCrory, P., Meeuwisse, W., Dvorak, J., Aubry, M., Bailes, J., Broglio, S., ... & Vos, P. E. (2017). Consensus statement on concussion in sport-the 5th international conference on concussion in sport held in Berlin, October 2016. British journal of sports medicine, 51(11), 838-847.

[37] Maas, A. I., Menon, D. K., Adelson, P. D., Andelic, N., Bell, M. J., Belli, A., ... & Schouten, J. (2017). Traumatic brain injury: integrated approaches to improve prevention, clinical care, and research. The Lancet Neurology, 16(12), 987-1048.

[38] Silverberg, N. D., & Iverson, G. L. (2011). Etiology of the post-concussion syndrome: Physiogenesis and psychogenesis revisited. NeuroRehabilitation, 29(4), 317-329.

[39] Lucas, S., Hoffman, J. M., Bell, K. R., & Dikmen, S. (2016). A prospective study of prevalence and characterization of headache following mild traumatic brain injury. Cephalalgia, 36(12), 1080-1087.

[40]Evans, R. W. (2006). Post-traumatic headaches. Neurology Clinics, 22(1), 237-249.

[41] Bendtsen, L., Jensen, R., & Olesen, J. (2010). Tension-type headache: An update on mechanisms and treatment. *Current Opinion in Neurology, 23*(3), 273-283.

[42] Ashina, H., Eigenbrodt, A. K., Seifert, T., Sinclair, A. J., Scher, A. I., Schytz, H. W., Lee, M. J., De Icco, R., Finkel, A. G., & Ashina, M. (2021). Post-traumatic headache attributed to traumatic brain injury: Classification, clinical characteristics, and treatment. The Lancet Neurology, 20(6), 460–469

[43] Smith, D. H., Johnson, V. E., & Stewart, W. (2018). Unraveling the pathophysiological threads linking brain injury and post-traumatic headaches. Acta Neuropsychologia, 35(5), 1231-1241.

[44] Lee, C., & Wang, D. (2020). Neurophysiological shifts after mild traumatic brain injury. Neurological Insights, 30(2), 134-145.

[45] Jones, A., Roberts, L., & Jackson, M. (2021). Impact of mTBI on sensory processing and headache. Journal of Headache Pain Management, 15(3), 215-228.

[46] Smith, D. (2019). Sleep patterns and recovery in traumatic brain injury. Neurorehabilitation & Neural Repair, 33(3), 203-211

[47] Johnson, C., & Lee, B. (2018). The relationship between stress and post-traumatic headaches. Journal of Headache & Pain Management, 15(2), 189-197

[48] American Migraine Foundation. (n.d.). Post-traumatic headache. Retrieved from https://americanmigrainefoundation.org/resource-library/post-traumatic-headache/.

[49] Williams, F., Brown, H., & Zhang, L. (2020). The role of hydration in headache prevention among TBI survivors. International Journal of Physiological and Pathological Research, 29(4), 333-341

[50] Ontario Neurotrauma Foundation. (2023). Guidelines for concussion/mTBI and persistent symptoms: Third edition. Retrieved from https://concussionsontario.org/sites/default/files/2023-03/Third_Edition.pdf.

[51] Smith, J. R., Brown, L. M., & Tew, K. K. (2020). The efficacy of pharmacological agents for post-traumatic headache management. Neurosurgical Updates, 88(3), 345-358.

[52] Martin, A. P., & Johnson, H. D. (2021). Cognitive-behavioral therapy: A cornerstone for managing chronic headaches. Psychology Today Review, 14(3), 120-139.

[53] Zhou, X., Weng, L., & Zhao, Q. (2022). Acupuncture as a therapeutic approach for headache management: An overview. Global Traditional Medicine Journal, 12(3), 110-127.

[54] Chambers, A. R., & Davis, B. L. (2019). Biofeedback as a preventative intervention for headache management. Journal of Headache and Pain Management, 156(2), 245-260.

[55] Thompson, N., & Greenberg, S. (2020). Integrating mindfulness practices into headache management: A review. Mind-Body Medicine, 29(4), 185-196.

[56] May, L. A., & Wilson, K. T. (2021). Sensory sensitivity and desensitization therapy among mTBI patients. Journal of Neuroscience and Rehabilitation, 42(5), 233-250.

[57] Silverberg, N. D., & Iverson, G. L. (2013). Etiology of the post-concussion syndrome: Physiogenesis and psychogenesis revisited. NeuroRehabilitation, 32(2), 329-338

[58] Schnurr, P. P., Lunney, C. A., & Sengupta, A. (2009). Posttraumatic stress disorder and head injury as risk factors for persistent post-concussive symptoms in veterans. Journal of Traumatic Stress, 22(6), 556-564.

[59] Evans, R. W., & Seifert, T. D. (2017). The role of the neurologist in treating concussion. Neurology Clinics, 35(3), 567-580.

[60] Langevin, H. M., & Sherman, K. J. (2007). Pathophysiological model for chronic low back pain integrating connective tissue and nervous system mechanisms. Medical Hypotheses, 68(1), 74-80.

[61] Gallai, V., Sarchielli, P., Genco, S., Alberti, A., & D'andrea, G. (2000). Chronic daily headache: biochemical and neurotransmitter abnormalities. *The Journal of Headache and Pain*, 1(3), 1-10. https://dx.doi.org/10.1007/s101940070031

[62] Frederiksen, S. D., Haanes, K., Warfvinge, K., & Edvinsson, L. (2017). Perivascular neurotransmitters: Regulation of cerebral blood flow and role in

primary headaches. *Journal of Cerebral Blood Flow & Metabolism*, 38(1), 1-12. https://dx.doi.org/10.1177/0271678X17747188

[63] Holland, P. R. (2009). Modulation of trigeminovascular processing: Novel insights into primary headache disorders. *Cephalalgia*, 29(12), 1221-1230. https://dx.doi.org/10.1177/03331024090290S302

[64] Samsam, M., Coveñas, R., Ahangari, R., & Yajeya, J. (2010). Neuropeptides and Other Chemical Mediators, and the Role of Anti-inflammatory Drugs in Primary Headaches. *Current Pharmaceutical Design*, 16(9), 1106-1120. https://dx.doi.org/10.2174/187152301 1009030170

[65] Dennis, E. L., & Disner, S. G. (2015). Neuroinflammation and Neuromodulation: Insights from Neuroimaging. *NeuroImage: Clinical*, 7, 276-286

[66] Edvinsson, L., & Uddman, R. (2005). Neurobiology in primary headaches. *Brain Research Reviews*, 48(3), 438-456. https://pubmed.ncbi.nlm.nih.gov/15914251/

[67] Borsook, D., Upadhyay, J., & Chudler, E. H. (2012). The Pain Elliptic: Mapping Circuits to Crack the Puzzle of Perception Pathways of Pain. *Current Opinion in Neurology, 25*(1), 43-49.

[68] Kim, J. H., Hoge, R. D., & Horovitz, S. G. (2013). Axonal injury mechanics and the manifestation of headaches post-TBI. NeuroTrauma Journal, 30(8), 567-575.

[69] Giza, C. C., & Hovda, D. A. (2014). The new neurometabolic cascade of concussion. Neurosurgery, 75(Suppl 4), S24–S33.

[70] Osborn, A. J., Mathias, J. L., & Fairweather-Schmidt, A. K. (2014). Depression following adult, non-penetrating traumatic brain injury: A meta-analysis examining methodological variables and sample characteristics. Neuroscience & Biobehavioral Reviews, 47, 1–15. https://psycnet.apa.org/record/2014-54170-002

Lucas, S. (2015). Headache management in concussion and mild traumatic brain injury. PM&R, 7(3 Suppl), S46–S53 Lamontagne, G., Belleville, G., Beaulieu-Bonneau, S., Souesme, G., Savard, J., Sirois, M.-J., Giguère, M., Tessier, D., Le Sage, N., & Ouellet, M.-C. (2021). Anxiety symptoms and disorders in the first year after sustaining mild traumatic brain injury. Rehabilitation Psychology. Advance online publication. https://doi.org/10.1037/rep0000422.

[71]Maleki et al. (2021) – *Post-traumatic Headache and Mild Traumatic Brain Injury: Brain Networks and Connectivity,* https://www.researchgate.net/publication/349833113

[72] Leung, A. (2020). Addressing chronic persistent headaches after MTBI as a neuropathic pain state. *The Journal of Headache and Pain,* 21, 113–120. https://doi.org/10.1186/s10194-020-01133-2

[73] Maleki et al. (2021). Post-traumatic headache and mild traumatic brain injury: Brain networks and connectivity. Retrieved from ResearchGate: https://www.researchgate.net/publication/349833113

[74] Olesen, J. (2018). The International Classification of Headache Disorders, 3rd edition. Cephalalgia, 38(1), 1–211.

[75]Bush, R. L., Yu, C. E., Povlishock, J. T., & Qin, Z. (2010). Time course of inflammation after traumatic brain injury. Experimental Neurology, 224(1), 82-89.

[76] Banks, W. A. (2016). From blood-brain barrier to blood-brain interface: new opportunities for CNS drug delivery. *Nature Reviews Drug Discovery,* 15(3), 183-204.

[77] However, in cases of mTBI or concussion, subtle axonal damage may go undetected by standard imaging. Advanced methods like Diffusion Tensor Imaging (DTI), a specialized form of MRI, can detect microstructural changes in white matter tracts, making it an invaluable tool in research and clinical settings for identifying axonal injuries in these cases.

[78] Smith, D. H., Shull, W. F., Huang, W., Xu, Y., Corwin, J. A., & King, J. M. (2003). Acute axonal injury in humans after traumatic brain injury. *The Journal of Neuroscience,* 23(19), 7750-7757.

[79] Bey, T., & Ostick, E. (2009). Serotonergic system in headache: potential therapeutic targets. *Current Opinion in Neurology,* 22(3), 229-234.

[80] Ashina, M., Goadsby, P. J., & Ziegler, D. (2017). The trigeminal nociceptive system and its role in primary headaches. The Journal of Headache and Pain, 18(1), 1-15.

[81] Menon, D. K. (2010). Central hormonal disturbances. In Clinical Neuroendocrinology. Cambridge University Press.

[82]Maskell, J., & Chisholm, K. (2014). Vestibular rehabilitation: a brief review. Current Neurology and Neuroscience Reports, 14(5), 413.

83 Alsalaheen, B. A., Mucha, A., Morris, L. O., Whitney, S. L., Furman, J. M., & Sparto, P. J. (2010). Vestibular rehabilitation for dizziness and balance disorders after concussion. *Journal of Neurologic Physical Therapy, 34*(2), 87–93. https://doi.org/10.1097/NPT.0b013e3181dde568

84 Hoffer, M. E., Balaban, C., Gottshall, K., Balough, B. J., Maddox, M. R., & Penta, J. R. (2017). Vestibular consequences of mild traumatic brain injury and blast exposure: A review. *Journal of Vestibular Research, 27*(2-3), 91–99. https://doi.org/10.3233/VES-170610

85 Varatharaj, A., & Galea, I. (2017). The systemic immune response to traumatic brain injury. Nature Reviews Neurology, 13(5), 229-242.

86 Bryant, R. A., Harvey, A. G., Burgess, J. R., & Collett, P. D. (2011). The association between post-traumatic stress disorder and headache in mild traumatic brain injury. Brain Injury, 25(7), 685-690

87 Maas, A. I. R., Stocchetti, N., & Bullock, R. (2017). Moderate and severe traumatic brain injury in adults. The Lancet Neurology, 16(12), 987-1048.

88 Viano, D. C., Ewing-Cobbs, L., & Carlson, M. C. (2005). Understanding the intricate relationship between traumatic brain injury and persistent headaches. Neuroscience Letters, 381(3), 185-189.

89 Davis, M. C., Moorthy, K. R., & Gaffney, D. J. (2017). Neurotransmitter systems in traumatic brain injury: Implications for headache. Journal of Headache and Pain, 18(1), 15.

90 Li F, Lu L, Shang S, Chen H, Wang P, Muthaiah VP, Yin X, Chen YC. (2021). Altered static and dynamic functional network connectivity in post-traumatic headache. Journal of Headache and Pain, 22(1), 137. https://pubmed.ncbi.nlm.nih.gov/34773973/

91 Miller, M. B., & Murphy, B. (2019). *Genetic factors in migraine and post-traumatic headache: Insights from recent studies.* Headache: The Journal of Head and Face Pain, 59(8), 1525-1535. https://doi.org/10.1111/head.13513

92 Hou, L., Han, X., Sheng, P., Tong, W., Li, Z., Xu, D., Yu, M., Huang, L., Zhao, Z., Lu, Y., & Dong, Y. (2013). *Risk factors associated with sleep disturbance following traumatic brain injury: clinical findings and questionnaire based study.* PLoS One, 8(10), e76087. https://doi.org/10.1371/journal.pone.0076087

93 Tanriverdi, F., De Bellis, A., Bizzarro, A., Sinisi, A. A., Bellastella, G., Pane, E., ... & Unluhizarci, K. (2015). Pituitary dysfunction after traumatic brain injury:

A clinical and pathophysiological approach. Endocrine Reviews, 36(3), 305–342. https://doi.org/10.1210/er.2014-1065

[94] Arzani, M., Jahromi, S.R., Ghorbani, Z., et al. (2020). Gut-brain Axis and migraine headache: a comprehensive review. *Journal of Headache and Pain*, 21, 15.

[95] Smith, A. (2020). Tailoring headache interventions through pattern recognition. *Clinical Neuroscience Review*, 12(1), 67-75.

[96] Johnson, T., & Welch, B. (2019). The role of digital tools in headache management. *Journal of Headache and Pain Management*, 15(3), 45-55.

[97] Kacerguis, M. C., & Schaffer, B. (2019). The role of headache diaries in chronic headache management: A review. Headache, 59(4), 500-511.

[98] Bjelland, I., Hartvigsen, G., & Østergaard, S. (2019). Triggers of migraine: An evidence-based approach. Headache, 59(3), 287-301

[99] Goldstein, R. Z., Nowak, D., & Cambron, J. C. (2015). The impact of smartphone applications on headache management: A systematic review. Headache, 55(5), 861-872

[100] Smith, A. (2020). Tailoring headache interventions through pattern recognition. Clinical Neuroscience Review, 12(1), 67–75;

Kacerguis, M. C., & Schaffer, B. (2019). The role of headache diaries in chronic headache management: A review. Headache, 59(4), 500–511.

[101] Lucas, S., Hoffman, J., Bell, K. R., & Dikmen, S. (2014). A prospective study of prevalence and characterization of headache following mild traumatic brain injury. Cephalalgia, 34(2), 93-102.

[102] Dodick, D. W. (2018). A Phase 2 randomized, double-blind, placebo-controlled trial of a CGRP inhibitor in the prevention of migraine. The Journal of Headache and Pain, 19, 65.

[103] Reddy, R. (2017). Cognitive-Behavioral Therapy for Post-Traumatic Headaches: A Randomized Controlled Trial. Journal of Headache and Pain Management, 10(3), 123-135.

[104] Goldstein, R. Z., Nowak, D., & Cambron, J. C. (2015). The impact of smartphone applications on headache management: A systematic review. Headache, 55(5), 861–872.

[105] Schürks, M., Kurth, T., & Buring, J. E. (2010). Genetic determinants of headache: Understanding inherited susceptibility as a key pathway to personalized pain management. *Nature Reviews Neurology*, 6(8), 434-441.

[106] Minen, M. T., Jalloh, A., Ortega, C. A., Powers, S., Sevick, M. A., & Lipton, R. B. (2016). User Experience with a Smartphone App to Track Headaches: Analysis of a Randomized Controlled Trial. Cephalalgia, 36(14), 1276–1287.

[107] Diener, H. C., & Charles, A. (2019). The changing management of migraine: from prophylaxis to precision treatment. Current Opinion in Neurology, 32(3), 427–434.

[108] Rains, J. C., Poceta, J. S., & Pollina, D. A. (2020). Cognitive behavioral treatment for sleep disorders in the primary care setting. Physiology & Behavior, 176, 139–148.

[109] Moldofsky, H., Custodio, H., & Veinot, K. (2017). Headaches and sleep disorders: A review of the literature. Journal of Neurological Research, 39(2), 123-134.

[110] O'Brien, L. M., & Kapur, V. K. (2022). Behavioral sleep interventions: Optimizing sleep in patients with headache disorders. Sleep Medicine Reviews, 61, 101559.

[111] Rains, J. C., Poceta, J. S., Hudgel, D. W., & Donn, S. M. (2015). Headache and sleep disorders: Review and clinical implications for headache management. Headache: The Journal of Head and Face Pain, 45(10), 1397-1406.

[112] Finan, P. H., Goodin, B. R., & Smith, M. T. (2013). The association of sleep and pain: An update and a path forward. The Journal of Pain, 14(12), 1539-1552.

[113] Tharanathan, K., James, T., Perera, M., Abhayaratne, M., & Goldstein, B. (2020). Circadian rhythm sleep-wake disorders and headache disorders: Pathophysiological and treatment implications. Sleep Medicine Reviews, 50, 101245.

[114] Rains, J. C. (2018). Sleep and headaches: A common association with important clinical implications. Headache: The Journal of Head and Face Pain, 58(7), 1074-1091.

[115] Chang, A. M., Aeschbach, D., Duffy, J. F., & Czeisler, C. A. (2015). Evening use of light-emitting eReaders negatively affects sleep, circadian timing, and next-morning alertness. Proceedings of the National Academy of Sciences, 112(4), 1232-1237

[116] Black, D. S., O'Reilly, G. A., Olmstead, R., Breen, E. C., & Irwin, M. R. (2015). Mindfulness meditation and improvement in sleep quality and daytime impairment among older adults with sleep disturbances: a randomized clinical trial. JAMA Internal Medicine, 175(4), 494-501.

[117] Revell, V. L., & Eastman, C. I. (2005). How to trick Mother Nature into letting you fly around or stay up all night. Journal of Biological Rhythms, 20(4), 353-365

[118] Brand, S., Gerber, M., Beck, J., Hatzinger, M., & Holsboer-Trachsler, E. (2010). Exercising, sleep-EEG patterns, and psychological functioning are related among adolescents. World Journal of Biological Psychiatry, 11(2), 129-140.

[119] Cheng, P., & Drake, C. (2016). Psychological and behavioral therapies for insomnia. Clinics in Chest Medicine, 37(4), 673-686

[120] Charles, A., & Brennan, K. C. (2009). The pathophysiology of migraine: Implications for treatment. Progress in Neurobiology, 87(2), 171-180. (Discusses inflammation in headaches and potential triggers.)

[121] Popkin, B. M., D'Anci, K. E., & Rosenberg, I. H. (2010). Water, hydration, and health. Nutrition Reviews, 68(8), 439-458.

[122] Mauskop, A., Varughese, J., & Vasquez, A. (2016). The role of magnesium in reducing the frequency of migraines. *Headache: The Journal of Head and Face Pain*, 56(6), 124-130.

[123] Lucas, M., Chocano-Bedoya, P., Shulze, M., Leitao, E., & Mirzaei, F. (2020). Inflammation and omega-3 fatty acids: A review of pathways and mechanisms of action. Nutritional Neuroscience, 23(6), 437-443.

[124] Mauskop, A., & Varughese, J. (2012). Why all migraine patients should be treated with magnesium. Journal of Neural Transmission, 119(5), 575-579.

[125] Boone, J. E., Tucker, L. A., Erickson, A. C., & Nielson, N. M. (2015). Vitamin B2 (riboflavin) intake and migraine prevention: A systematic review. Headache: The Journal of Head and Face Pain, 55(7), 1156-1161

[126] Popkin, B. M., D'Anci, K. E., & Rosenberg, I. H. (2010). Water, hydration, and health. Nutrition Reviews, 68(8), 439-458., used before.

[127] Larsen, F. J., et al. (2014). Dietary nitrate and headache: A review of vascular effects. Journal of Headache and Pain, 15(1), 1–9.

[128] Lipton, R. B., Newman, L. C., Cohen, J. S., & Solomon, S. (1989). Aspartame as a dietary trigger of headache. Headache, 29(2), 90-92.

[129] Hoffmann, T. K., (2006). Histamine intolerance and mast cell activation – Diseases of increasing significance. Acta Clinica Croatica. 45(1), 49-58

[130] Lipton, R. B., Bigal, M. E., Diamond, M., Freitag, F., Reed, M. L., & Stewart, W. F. (2014). Migraine prevalence, disease burden, and the need for preventive therapy. Neurology, 68(5), 343-349.

[131] Sawka, M. N., Cheuvront, S. N., & Carter, R. (2005). Human water needs. Nutrition Reviews, 63(6), S30-S39.

[132] Institute of Medicine. (2004). Dietary Reference Intakes for Water, Potassium, Sodium, Chloride, and Sulfate. National Academies Press.

[133] Maughan, R. J. (2003). Impact of mild dehydration on wellness and on exercise performance. European Journal of Clinical Nutrition, 57(S2), S19-S23.

[134] Mauskop, A., & Varughese, J. (2022). The role of magnesium in the pathogenesis and treatment of migraines. *Clinics in Headache*, *12*(3), 123-134.

[135] Thompson, E., Loder, E., Lin, W.-Y., Ridenour, T., & Cheng, K.-L. (2020). Efficacy of riboflavin (vitamin B2) as a prophylaxis in students with migraines. *Neurology and Therapy*, *9*(1), 183-193.

[136] Ramsden, C. E., Faurot, K. R., Zamora, D., Suchindran, C. M., Ringel, A., & Hibbeln, J. R. (2013). An anti-inflammatory diet as treatment for headache: A randomized controlled crossover trial. *Journal of Headache and Pain Management*, *10*(2), 153–165.

[137] Sándor, P. S., Afra, J., Ambrosini, A., Schoenen, J., & Ferrari, M. D. (2019). Prophylactic treatment of migraine with Coenzyme Q10: A placebo-controlled randomized double-blind 3-month trial. *Cephalalgia*, *30*(3), 298-306.

[138] Goyal, M., Singh, S., Sibinga, E. M., Gould, N. F., Rowland-Seymour, A., Sharma, R., ... & Haythornthwaite, J. A. (2014). Meditation Programs for Psychological Stress and Well-being: A Systematic Review and Meta-analysis. JAMA Internal Medicine, 174(3), 357-368.

[139] Zeidan, F., Martucci, K. T., Kraft, R. A., McHaffie, J. G., & Coghill, R. C. (2015). Neural correlates of mindfulness meditation-related anxiety relief. Social Cognitive and Affective Neuroscience, 9(6), 751–759.

[140] Lennington, J. B., & Goulet, M. (2016). The relationships between psychological factors and post-traumatic headache after mild traumatic brain injury: A scoping review. The Clinical Journal of Pain, 32(12), 1014-1025.

[141] Stocchetti, N., & Zanier, E. R. (2016). Chronic impact of traumatic brain injury on outcome and quality of life: A narrative review. Critical Care, 20(1), 148

[142] Nestoriuc, Y., & Martin, A. (2007). Efficacy of biofeedback for migraine: A meta-analysis. Pain, 128(1-2), 111-127. https://doi.org/10.1016/j.pain.2006.09.007

[143] Zeidan, F., Martucci, K. T., Kraft, R. A., McHaffie, J. G., & Coghill, R. C. (2015). Neural correlates of mindfulness meditation-related anxiety relief. Social Cognitive and Affective Neuroscience, 9(6), 751-759.

[144] Werner, J. K., & Collen, J. F. (2019). Mindfulness-Based Stress Reduction as a Treatment for Chronic Insomnia in Traumatic Brain Injury Patients. *Sleep*, 42(Supplement 1), A158. Retrieved from https://dx.doi.org/10.1093/SLEEP/ZSZ067.390.

[145] Goyal, M., Singh, S., Sibinga, E. M., Gould, N. F., Rowland-Seymour, A., Sharma, R., ... & Haythornthwaite, J. A. (2014). Meditation Programs for Psychological Stress and Well-being: A Systematic Review and Meta-analysis. *JAMA Internal Medicine*, 174(3), 357-368.

[146] Conway, J., Brittain, K., & Trenholm, K. (2015). Progressive Muscle Relaxation: Efficacy for Reducing Headache Intensity. Clinical Pain Journal, 32(5), 341-345

[147] Kabat-Zinn, J. (2005) Chapter 4. Coming to Our Senses: Healing Ourselves and the World Through Mindfulness. New York, NY: Hyperion. This book delves into the application of mindfulness practices, including progressive muscle relaxation and deep breathing techniques, for stress reduction and overall well-being. It provides comprehensive insights into how these methods can be integrated into daily life to manage stress effectively. Chapter 4, titled "Embracing Formal Practice: Tasting Mindfulness" delves into various mindfulness practices, including those techniques, and their applications in stress reduction.

[148] Davidson, R. J., & Lutz, A. (2008). Buddha's brain: Neuroplasticity and meditation. IEEE Signal Processing Magazine, 25(1), 176-174. https://doi.org/10.1109/MSP.2008.4431873

[149] Jensen, M. P. (2011). Psychosocial approaches to pain management: An organizational framework. *Pain, 152*(3), S2-S8. https://doi.org/10.1016/j.pain.2010.09.002

[150] Leddy, J. J., Cox, J. L., & Baker, J. G. (2012). Exercise treatment for concussion. Current Sports Medicine Reports, 11(6), 321-32.: This study discusses the benefits of exercise in concussion management, highlighting how physical activity can promote better blood flow and stimulate the release of endorphins, which act as natural painkillers. https://ubortho.com/wp-content/uploads/2015/04/leddyconcussion.pdf

[151] Smith, R. & Jones, T. (2019). The Importance of Multidisciplinary Teams in Treating Brain Injury-Related Headaches. Clinical Neurology Review, 45(7), 780-785. This article underscores the importance of multidisciplinary approaches in treating brain injury-related headaches, noting that regular physical activity enhances mood and facilitates stress reduction, key factors in minimizing headache occurrences.

[152] Brown, S., Miller, T., & Davis, P. (2020). Guidelines for exercise in post-concussion recovery. The Clinical Journal of Sports Medicine, 30(7), 557-563. This paper provides guidelines for exercise in post-concussion recovery, emphasizing the necessity of balancing exercise intensity to prevent overexertion and recommending gradual progression under healthcare professional guidance.

[153] Silverberg, N. D., & Iverson, G. L. (2013). Is rest after concussion "the best medicine?": Recommendations for activity resumption following concussion in athletes, civilians, and military service members. *Journal of Head Trauma Rehabilitation, 28*(4), 250-259. https://doi.org/10.1097/HTR.0b013e31825ad658

[154] Mucha, A., Collins, M. W., Elbin, R., Furman, J. M., Troutman-Enseki, C., & DeWolf, R. M. (2014). A brief vestibular and ocular motor examination (VOME) differentiates concussion from common medical conditions. *American Journal of Sports Medicine, 42*(4), 963-971. https://doi.org/10.1177/0363546514543775

[155] Chio, CC., Lin, HJ., Tian, YF. et al. Exercise attenuates neurological deficits by stimulating a critical HSP70/NF-κB/IL-6/synapsin I axis in traumatic brain injury rats. J Neuroinflammation 14, 90 (2017). https://doi.org/10.1186/s12974-017-0867-9

[156] Dishman, R.K., et al., (2015). Endorphins and exercise. Sports Medicine, 45(10), 1391-1405

[157] Erickson, K.I., & Voss, M.W. (2013). Exercise effects on brain and cognition across age groups. Journal of Neuroscience, 33(47), 17685-17695

158 Kredlow, M. A., Capozzoli, M. C., Hearon, B. A., Calkins, A. W., & Otto, M. W. (2015). The effects of physical activity on sleep: A meta-analytic review. Journal of Behavioral Medicine, 38(3), 427–449. https://doi.org/10.1007/s10865-015-9617-6

159 Giza, C. C., & Hovda, D. A. (2014). The neurometabolic cascade of concussion. Journal of Athletic Training provides a comprehensive overview of the pathophysiological processes that occur following a concussion., 49(1), 141-155. https://doi.org/10.4085/1062-6050-49.1.15

160 Leddy, J. J., Haider, M. N., Ellis, M. J., & Willer, B. S. (2018). "Exercise is medicine for concussion." Current Sports Medicine Reports, 17(8), 262-270. https://doi.org/10.1249/JSR.0000000000000505

161 UPMC Sports Medicine Concussion Program. (2016). *UPMC 5-stage concussion rehab protocol.* Retrieved from https://macconcussion.com/wp-content/uploads/2016/08/UPMC-5-Stage-Concussion-Rehab-Protocol.pdf

162 McCrory, P., Meeuwisse, W., Dvorak, J., Aubry, M., Bailes, J., Broglio, S., … & Vos, P. E. (2017). Consensus statement on concussion in sport: The 5th International Conference on Concussion in Sport held in Berlin, October 2016. British Journal of Sports Medicine, 51(11), 838–847. https://doi.org/10.1136/bjsports-2017-097699

163 Lucas, S. (2014). Headache management in concussion and mild traumatic brain injury. PM&R, 6(10 Suppl 2), S406–S412. https://doi.org/10.1016/j.pmrj.2014.08.015 ;Ashina, M., et al. (2021). CGRP-targeted therapies for migraine: A review of clinical evidence and future directions. Nature Reviews Neurology, 17(7), 421–432. https://doi.org/10.1038/s41582-021-00521-5

164 Johnson, L., & Taylor, M. (2019). The role of physical therapy in managing post-traumatic headaches. Physical Therapy in Sport, 35, 65-72.

165 Brown, A. (2021). Alternative therapies in headache management. Journal of Integrative Medicine, 19(3), 120-128.; Nestoriuc, Y., & Martin, A. (2007). Efficacy of biofeedback for migraine: A meta-analysis. Pain, 128(1–2), 111–127. https://doi.org/10.1016/j.pain.2006.09.007

166 Bigal, M. E., Lipton, R. B. (2009). Overuse of acute migraine medications and migraine progression. *Current Pain and Headache Reports, 13*(1), 39-43. https://doi.org/10.1007/s11916-009-0048-3

[167] Silberstein, S. D. (2004). Migraine. *The Lancet, 363*(9406), 381-391. https://doi.org/10.1016/S0140-6736(04)15440-8

[168] Dodick, D. W., & Silberstein, S. D. (2006). "Central Sensitization Theory of Migraine: Clinical Implications". *Headache: The Journal of Head and Face Pain, 46*(Suppl 4), S182-S191. https://doi.org/10.1111/j.1526-4610.2006.00602.x

[169] Holroyd, C. A., Cottrell, S., O'Donnell, F. J., MacGregor, B. A., & Smith, J. W. (2009). Beta-blockers for the prevention of migraines in adults. Journal of Neurology, Neurosurgery & Psychiatry, 80(5), 123–130.

[170] Silberstein, S. D. (2015). Preventive migraine treatment. *Continuum: Lifelong Learning in Neurology, 21*(4, Headache), 973-989. https://doi.org/10.1212/CON.0000000000000199

[171] Zirovich, M. D., Pangarkar, S., Manh, C., Chen, L., Vangala, S., & Izuchukwu, I. S. (2021). Botulinum Toxin Type A for the Treatment of Post-traumatic Headache: A Randomized, Placebo-Controlled, Cross-over Study. *Military Medicine, 186*(5-6), 493-499. https://doi.org/10.1093/milmed/usaa391

[172] Edvinsson, L., Haanes, K. A., Warfvinge, K., & Krause, D. N. (2018). CGRP as the target of new migraine therapies—successful translation from bench to clinic. Nature Reviews Neurology, 14(6), 338-350. https://doi.org/10.1038/s41582-018-0003-1

[173] Pomes, L., Guglielmetti, M., Bertamino, E., Simmaco, M., Borro, M., & Martelletti, P. (2019). Optimising migraine treatment: from drug-drug interactions to personalized medicine. Journal of Headache and Pain, 20(1), 56 https://doi.org/10.1186/s10194-019-1010-3

[174] Rizzoli, P. (2012). Preventive pharmacotherapy in five steps: Thoughts for a new treatment paradigm. Neurology, 78(IS), S15-S24.

[175] Fernández-de-las-Peñas, C., Ge, H. Y., Arendt-Nielsen, L., Cuadrado, M. L., & Pareja, J. A. (2007). Myofascial trigger points and sensitization: An updated pain model for tension-type headache. Cephalalgia, 27(4), 383–393. https://journals.sagepub.com/doi/pdf/10.1111/j.1468-2982.2007.01295.x?utm_source=copilot.com

[176] Biondi, D. M. (2005). Physical treatments for headache: A structured review. Headache: The Journal of Head and Face Pain, 45(4), 738-746.

[177] Vickers, A. J., Cronin, A. M., Maschino, A. C., Lewith, G., MacPherson, H., Foster, N. E., Sherman, K. J., & Witt, C. M. (2012). Acupuncture for Chronic

Pain: Individual Patient Data Meta-analysis. Archives of Internal Medicine, 172(19), 1444-1453. https://doi.org/10.1001/archinternmed.2012.3654

[178] Bryans, R., Decina, P., Descarreaux, M., Duranleau, M., Marcoux, H., Potter, B., Ruegg, R., Shaw, L., Watkin, R., & White, E. (2011). Evidence-based guidelines for the chiropractic treatment of adults with headache. The Journal of the Canadian Chiropractic Association, 55(2), 100-112. https://doi.org/10.1016/j.jmpt.2011.01.001

[179] Nestoriuc, Y., & Martin, A. (2007). Efficacy of biofeedback for migraine: A meta-analysis. Pain, 128(1-2), 111-127. https://doi.org/10.1016/j.pain.2006.09.007

[180] Van Dam, N. T., van Vugt, M. K., Vago, D. R., Schmalzl, L., Saron, C. D., Olendzki, A., Meissner, T., Lazar, S. W., Kerr, C. E., Gorchov, J., Fox, K. C. R., Field, B. A., Britton, W. B., Brefczynski-Lewis, J. A., & Meyer, D. E. (2018). Mind the hype: A critical evaluation and prescriptive agenda for research on mindfulness and meditation. Perspectives on Psychological Science, 13(1), 36-61. https://doi.org/10.1177/1745691617709589

[181] Gaul, C., Visscher, C. M., Bhola, R., Sorbi, M. J., Galli, F., Rasmussen, A. V., & Jensen, R. (2011). Team players against headache: multidisciplinary treatment of primary headaches and medication overuse headache. The Journal of Headache and Pain, 12(5), 511–519. https://doi.org/10.1007/s10194-011-0364-y

[182] Linde, K., Allais, G., Brinkhaus, B., Manheimer, E., Vickers, A., & White, A. (2009). Non-pharmacological treatments for migraine and tension-type headache: A systematic review. The Cochrane Database of Systematic Reviews, 2009(1), CD001218. https://doi.org/10.1002/14651858.CD001218.pub2

[183] Brown, A. R., & Donahue, P. (2021). Family Involvement and Headache Management: The Role of Social Support Systems. Journal of Neurology Case Studies, 12(4), 233-240.

[184] Smith, A., Thompson, L., & Green, H. (2021). The role of routine and triggers in headache management. Neuroscience in Practice, 15(4), 102-115

[185] Brown, T., & White, J. (2019). Creating supportive environments for recovery. Journal of Traumatic Brain Injury, 12(3), 45-58.

[186] Johnson, R. (2020). Lifestyle adaptations for headache prevention after brain injury. Clinical Rehabilitation, 28(7), 78-89.

[187] Smith, R. A., Taylor, P., & Johnson, C. (2020). A comprehensive approach to headache management for TBI survivors. Brain Injury Solutions Journal, 33(8), 1023-1035.

[188] Brown, T., & Green, J. (2019). The role of consistent sleep patterns in headache prevention. It highlights the importance of maintaining regular sleep schedules to reduce the frequency and intensity of headaches. The research suggests that disruptions in sleep patterns can trigger headaches and that establishing consistent sleep routines can be an effective preventive measure. Journal of Neurological Research, 45(3), 230-242.

[189] Johnson, L., Xiao, M., & Thompson, H. (2021). Nutritional strategies for headache management in traumatic brain injury. *Nutrition and Brain Health*, 12(2), 107-118

[190] Lew, H. L., et al. (2009). Sensory and cognitive dysfunction after blast-related mild traumatic brain injury. Journal of Rehabilitation Research & Development

[191] Zebenholzer, K., Gall, W., & Wöber, C. (2011). Migraine and risk factors of migraine. Wiener Medizinische Wochenschrift, 161(11-12), 286-290. doi:10.1007/s10354-011-0024-x

[192] Holroyd, K. A., & Lipchik, G. L. (1999). The impact of functional impairment: Evidence for a biopsychosocial model. Headache: The Journal of Head and Face Pain, 39(7), 474-482.

[193] Rains, J. C., & Poceta, J. S. (2010). Headache and sleep disorders: Review and clinical implications. Headache: The Journal of Head and Face Pain, 50(7), 1170–1179

[194] Lew, H. L., Poole, J. H., Guillory, S. B., Salerno, R. M., & Leskin, G. A. (2009). Sensory and cognitive dysfunction after blast-related mild traumatic brain injury. Journal of Rehabilitation Research & Development, 46(6), 757–776.

[195] Jensen, M. P. (2011). Psychosocial approaches to pain management: An organizational framework. Pain, 152(3), S2–S8.

[196] Association for Behavioral and Cognitive Therapies. (n.d.). Adult traumatic brain injury for supporters of individuals with traumatic brain injury. Retrieved from https://www.abct.org/fact-sheets/adult-traumatic-brain-injury-for-supporters-of-individuals-with-traumatic-brain-injury/

[197] Sapolsky, R. M. (2004). Why zebras don't get ulcers: The acclaimed guide to stress, stress-related diseases, and coping. New York: Henry Holt and Company.

[198] CT Brain Injury (2023). Effective Communication Strategies for Families Affected by Traumatic Brain Injury (TBI). Retrieved from https://www.ctbraininjury.com/post/effective-communication-strategies-for-families-affected-by-traumatic-brain-injury-tbi

[199] Berkman, L. F., Glass, T., Brissette, I., & Seeman, T. E. (2000). From social integration to health: Durkheim in the new millennium. Social Science & Medicine, 51(6), 843-857.

[200] Starcevic, V. (2017). Cyber-chondria: Challenges of problematic online searches for health-related information. Psychotherapy and Psychosomatics, 86(3), 129-133

[201] Raj, R. et al. (2020). The effect of professional support on outcomes for people affected by traumatic brain injury: A systematic review. Disability and Rehabilitation, 42(17), 2442-2452.

[202] Ponsford, J. et al. (2014). Long-term outcomes following traumatic brain injury: A comparative analysis of survivors. Journal of Rehabilitation Medicine, 46(7), 578-585.

[203] World Health Organization. (2021). Neurological disorders: Public health challenges. WHO Press; Sandel, M. E., Wright, J., & Peele, B. (2020). Management of headache after brain injury. Journal of Head Trauma Rehabilitation, 35(1), 3-13.

[204] Mason, R., Miller, J., & Scott, A. (2022). Impact of sleep on recovery post-traumatic brain injury. Journal of Neurotrauma, 39(3), 201-210

[205] Ouellet, M.-C., & Morin, C. M. (2006). Subjective and objective measures of insomnia in the context of traumatic brain injury. Journal of Head Trauma Rehabilitation, 21(6), 502–516; Edinger, J. D., & Means, M. K. (2005). CBT-I as a treatment for primary insomnia: A meta-analysis. Sleep, 28(6), 603–614.

[206] Brown, T., & Taylor, S. (2020). Nutrition and headache management post-concussion. Nutrition Reviews, 78(5), 401-409.

[207] Clark, N., Taylor, P., & White, R. (2021). The role of supplements in headache prevention. Headache: The Journal of Head and Face Pain, 61(10), 850-857

[208] Leddy, J. J., Haider, M. N., Ellis, M. J., & Willer, B. S. (2018). Exercise is medicine for concussion. Current Sports Medicine Reports, 17(8), 262–270.

[209] Turner, H., & Miller, T. (2021). Balancing physical activity levels in TBI recovery. Journal of Head Trauma Rehabilitation, 36(2), 90-95.

[210] Anderson, R., Stevens, G., & King, J. (2022). Stress management strategies for post-traumatic headache reduction. Behavioral Neuroscience, 136(6), 594-602

Sauro, K. M., & Becker, W. J. (2009). The stress and migraine interaction. Headache, 49(9), 1378–1386.

Wells, R. E., O'Connell, N., Pierce, C. R., et al. (2014). Mindfulness meditation for migraines: A pilot randomized controlled trial. Headache, 54(9), 1484–1495.; Nestoriuc, Y., & Martin, A. (2007). Efficacy of biofeedback for migraine: A meta-analysis. Pain, 128(1–2), 111–127.

[211] Martin, P. R., & MacLeod, C. (2009). Behavioral management of headache triggers: Avoidance of triggers is an inadequate strategy. Clinical Psychology Review, 29(6), 483–495.

[212] Leddy, J. J., Baker, J. G., & Willer, B. (2016). Active rehabilitation of concussion and post-concussion syndrome. Physical Medicine and Rehabilitation Clinics of North America, 27(2), 437–454

[213] Hoffmann, J., & Recober, A. (2013). Nutritional and metabolic aspects of migraine management. Continuum, 19(4), 1043–1057.; Schoenen, J., Jacquy, J., & Lenaerts, M. (1998). Effectiveness of high-dose riboflavin in migraine prophylaxis. Neurology, 50(2), 466–470.

[214] Ouellet, M.-C., & Morin, C. M. (2006). Subjective and objective measures of insomnia in the context of traumatic brain injury. Journal of Head Trauma Rehabilitation, 21(6), 502–516.

[215] Wells, R. E., O'Connell, N., Pierce, C. R., et al. (2014). Mindfulness meditation for migraines: A pilot randomized controlled trial. Headache, 54(9), 1484–1495.

[216] Linde, K., Allais, G., Brinkhaus, B., et al. (2016). Acupuncture for the prevention of tension-type headache. Cochrane Database of Systematic Reviews, 4, CD007587.; Nestoriuc, Y., & Martin, A. (2007). Efficacy of biofeedback for migraine: A meta-analysis. Pain, 128(1–2), 111–127.

[217] Martin, P. R., & MacLeod, C. (2009). Behavioral management of headache triggers: Avoidance of triggers is an inadequate strategy. Clinical Psychology Review, 29(6), 483–495.

[218] Sturgeon, J. A., & Zautra, A. J. (2010). Resilience: A new paradigm for adaptation to chronic pain. Current Pain and Headache Reports, 14(2), 105–112.

[219] Buse, D. C., et al. (2019). Use of technology in migraine management: A review of mobile apps and wearables. Headache, 59(7), 1137–1154

[220] Sandel, M. E., Wright, J., & Peele, B. (2020). Management of headache after brain injury. Journal of Head Trauma Rehabilitation, 35(1), 3–13

[221] Jensen, M. P., & Turk, D. C. (2014). Contributions of psychology to the understanding and treatment of people with chronic pain. American Psychologist, 69(2), 105–118.

[222] Grossman, P., Niemann, L., Schmidt, S., & Walach, H. (2004). Mindfulness-based stress reduction and health benefits: A meta-analysis. Journal of Psychosomatic Research, 57(1), 35–43

[223] Mauskop, A., & Sun-Edelstein, C. (2009). Dietary factors and triggers in migraine. Current Pain and Headache Reports, 13(6), 413–419

[224] Linde, M., et al. (2013). Headache management and quality of life: A systematic review. Cephalalgia, 33(9), 629–642.

[225] Hoge, C. W., Goldberg, H. M., & Castro, C. A. (2008). Care of war veterans with mild traumatic brain injury—flawed perspectives. New England Journal of Medicine, 358(16), 1585–1587.

[226] Lucas, S., Hoffman, J. M., Bell, K. R., & Dikmen, S. (2012). A prospective study of prevalence and characterization of headache following mild traumatic brain injury. Cephalalgia, 32(5), 398–402.

[227] Iverson, G. L., & Lange, R. T. (2011). Post-concussion syndrome. In M. R. Schoenberg & J. G. Scott (Eds.), The Little Black Book of Neuropsychology. Springer.

[228] CDC. (2018). Heads Up: Brain Injury in Your Practice. Centers for Disease Control and Prevention

[229] Hoffmann, J., & Recober, A. (2013).Nutritional and metabolic aspects of migraine management. Continuum, 19(4), 1043–1057.

[230] Ouellet, M.-C., & Morin, C. M. (2006). Insomnia following traumatic brain injury. Journal of Head Trauma Rehabilitation, 21(6), 502–516.

[231] Buse, D. C., et al. (2019). Use of technology in migraine management: A review of mobile apps and wearables. Headache, 59(7), 1137–1154.